D0873842

helping
deaf
and
hard of hearing
students
to use
SPOKEN LANGUAGE

*We dedicate this book to the many children with hearing loss and their families
who have shaped our knowledge and experiences with
spoken language development, and to the teachers
who work tirelessly for their students.*

*We also dedicate this book to our families, who give us all their
support and love. They are: Amy, Bryan, Dewey, and William.*

helping
deaf
and
hard of hearing
students
to use
SPOKEN
LANGUAGE

A GUIDE FOR EDUCATORS AND FAMILIES

SUSAN R. EASTERBROOKS
ELLEN L. ESTES

Foreword by Mary Ellen Nevins

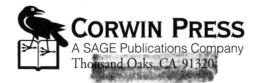

CORWIN PRESS
A SAGE Publications Company
Thousand Oaks, CA 91320

For information:

Corwin Press
A Sage Publications Company
2455 Teller Road
Thousand Oaks, California 91320
www.corwinpress.com

Sage Publications Ltd.
1 Oliver's Yard
55 City Road
London, EC1Y 1SP
United Kingdom

Sage Publications India Pvt. Ltd.
B 1/I 1 Mohan Cooperative Industrial Area
Mathura Road, New Delhi 110 044
India

Sage Publications Asia-Pacific Pte. Ltd.
33 Pekin Street #02-01
Far East Square
Singapore 048763

Printed in the United States of America

Library of Congress Cataloging-in-Publication Data

Easterbrooks, Susan R.
Helping deaf and hard of hearing students to use spoken language: a guide for educators and families/Susan R. Easterbrooks and Ellen L. Estes.
   p. cm.
Includes bibliographical references (p.   ) and index.
ISBN 978-1-4129-2732-1 (cloth)
ISBN 978-1-4129-2733-8 (pbk.)
   1. Deaf children—Language. 2. Hearing impaired children—Language.
3. Deaf children—Education. 4. Hearing impaired children—Education.
I. Estes, Ellen L. II. Title.

HV2483.E23 2007
371.91'24622—dc22   2006102697

This book is printed on acid-free paper.

07   08   09   10   11   10   9   8   7   6   5   4   3   2   1

Acquisitions Editor:	Allyson P. Sharp
Editorial Assistant:	Nadia Kashper
Production Editor:	Laureen A. Shea
Typesetter:	C&M Digitals (P) Ltd.
Proofreader:	Dorothy Hoffman
Indexer:	Kathy Paparchontis
Cover Designer:	Michael Dubowe
Graphic Designer:	Lisa Miller

Contents

Foreword

Mary Ellen Nevins, EdD
Teacher, Teacher Educator, Author, Educational Consultant,
and Professional Development Specialist
Currently in Private Practice in Tecumseh, MI

Articulate and coherent communication skills in the language of the majority allow the individual who possesses them to more easily negotiate the world in which he or she lives. This is especially evident in the experiences of individuals born with significant hearing loss. Children who are deaf or hard of hearing are at a considerable disadvantage in learning to talk if they do not hear clearly enough to perceive the nuances of sound that make up spoken language.

Limitations of hearing aids available in the past created very real barriers to the acquisition of spoken language. Historically, efforts to develop spoken language in deaf children were met with more than occasional success. However, the enormity of the task often left children with such limited spoken language competence that they could communicate only with immediate family, teachers, and close family friends.

In years past, educators became specially trained and prepared to undertake this challenging task. Not surprisingly, the global advances in technology that have influenced our everyday lives have created opportunities for a new generation of deaf children to learn spoken language more easily by mitigating the effects of severe to profound hearing loss. Today's digital hearing aids and cochlear implants have provided unprecedented auditory access for the children who receive these devices. There are children for whom these devices are all they need to acquire spoken language; however, there remain a significant number of children with hearing loss who will require more from the teachers and clinicians with whom they work.

These are children who perhaps come to language learning somewhat later in life or who are challenged by processing or learning issues beyond the peripheral hearing loss. Auditory access alone, even with intentional guidance by the teacher and clinician, will not be sufficient for the acquisition of spoken language. These children will need more intentional instruction to launch their journey in spoken language learning. And, once underway, they will continue to benefit from the systematic application of the knowledge and skills involved in this instruction.

It is our good fortune that authors Susan Easterbrooks and Ellen Estes have teamed up to create a text designed to assist teachers and speech and hearing professionals in developing spoken language in children with hearing loss. Geared specifically for the child for whom auditory access is not sufficient for language acquisition without intentional instruction, this text will be of particular benefit to the teacher or clinician working with a child who presents as "languageless."

The authors' combination of theory and practice in this book encourages novice teachers and speech-language pathologists to create a conceptual framework for the task of developing spoken language intentionally. At the same time it provides rich and practical examples of objectives that will lead to a child's learning to talk. Just as a fledgling artist learns concepts of figure, ground, distance, and perspective as a prelude to drawing and painting, so too the novice speech and hearing professional will be exposed to concepts such as auditory brain tasks, listening and speaking skills, and external factors that will influence teaching and learning. Once armed with the conceptual framework, the reader is challenged to locate the intersection of these factors that represents the point at which any particular student stands in the journey to spoken language competence. The varying model aspects can be manipulated to assist the child in moving through the three dimensions of spoken language learning.

Susan and Ellen are to be commended for their thoughtful preparation of this text. The accessibility of the concepts presented through their framework will allow for precise communication between and among all those helping the child. As expert teachers of children with hearing loss and as experienced teacher educators, the authors demonstrate their own scientific knowledge and artistic skill in crafting this text to invite us to learn more about developing spoken language in children with hearing loss.

Preface

The ability to communicate with others develops normally and naturally for most young children unless something out of the ordinary occurs. A hearing loss is one of those out of the ordinary events that can make it difficult for children to learn to communicate. Spoken language is a very complicated task requiring our amazing brains to act as master coordinators of thoughts, sounds, and movements in what appears to be an effortless process. A hearing loss influences communication development. One tool we have for overcoming these influences is a well-prepared teacher. Another tool is an empowered parent. Finally, technological advances have made it more likely that children who are deaf and hard of hearing will hear well enough to develop spoken language. This book was written for the teachers who are in the important position of working with children who have hearing losses, whether they are regular educators, special educators, early interventionists, or specially trained teachers of children who are deaf or hard of hearing. How you have come to be working with a deaf or hard of hearing child does not matter. What you can do about it does.

In this book, we focus specifically on young children who are learning spoken language and not sign language. American Sign Language (ASL) is a wonderful language that provides many deaf children with options to communicate richly and completely; however, it is not the focus of this book (for a comprehensive discussion of learning a signed language, see Easterbrooks and Baker, 2002).

There is an art and a science to imparting spoken language to children who are deaf or hard of hearing. The art comes in the creative ways we interact with a child to support the development of communication. In Part 1 of this book, you will learn numerous strategies for teaching spoken communication. We hope you will apply these artfully. There is also a science to intervening with deaf and hard of hearing children. In Part 2 you will learn about the science behind the art of teaching spoken communication to children who are deaf and hard of hearing. The better one understands the science, the better an artist he or she can become.

Acknowledgments

No book of this nature is written without significant advice and support from friends and colleagues. Contributions of editing, artwork, and other graphics and special content are found on most pages.

We are indebted to the many individuals who read and reread various versions of the chapters, each time making suggestions that helped both focus and flow. Although we have tried to recall all those who contributed, we must apologize to those we missed. Please know that your contribution is equally valued. We thank the following individuals (in alphabetical order) for reading and making comments on different chapters along the way: Shelley Carr, Leslie Doster, Cheryl Easterbrooks, Janet Felice, Katie Huffstutler, Jane Kassing, Deborah Knight, Judy Kroese, Karen Kupper, Linda Lasker, Kacey Lindgren, Melissa McDonald, Beth Miller, Mary Ellen Nevins, Christine O'Connor, Marion Oliver, Jessica Page, Julie Pepper, Janice Rice, and Lucia Villahoz. We thank the board of directors, administrators, faculty, and staff of the Katherine Hamm Center of the Atlanta Speech School for their additional support to us during the writing process. We also extend special thanks to Dr. Norman P. Erber, Rehabilitation Consultant, Helosonics/Clavis Publishing, whose multiple readings of the chapters were invaluable in shaping much of the information presented.

We wish to thank several individuals for their contributions of pictures, graphics, and other visual tools. We thank James Poulakos and Moustafa Elsaway of Georgia State University's Digital Café, for their rendering of the *Model of Auditory, Speech, and Language Development* in Chapter 1. Mr. Poulakos also contributed additional graphics including the articulation, phonation, resonation, thought, and language graphics. We thank Jack Zimmermann, the photographer who took many of the photos in the book, and Ellen Estes, who designed and crafted many of the charts and graphs in the book. We also thank Brad Ingrao (www.e-audiology.net), who modified his *Audiogram of Speech Sounds* to meet the needs of this book.

Several organizations and vendors also graciously permitted us to use their materials. Table 1.2 and Figures 6.1, 6.7, and 6.13 come from *The Speech Chain: The Physics and Biology of Spoken Language* (Denes & Pinson, 1993). We thank Natus® Medical Incorporated for the use of their pictures of infant hearing screening. We thank Gallaudet University for permission to reprint their Schematic of the Outer, Middle, and Inner Ear with Auditory Nerve (source: http://clerccenter.gallaudet.edu/InfoToGo/535/ear.gif, downloaded March 25, 2006). We acknowledge the Inspiration Corporation, whose software was used to create the word wheel at the end of Chapter 5, and www.clipart.com, whose subscription allowed us to download the images of cubes and books.

Finally, we extend special thanks to Ellen Rhoades, Certified Auditory Verbal Therapist (www.auditoryverbaltraining.com), who graciously revised her *Learning to Listen Sounds* to develop Resource C, *Sound-Object Associations.* This is an invaluable contribution to the teachers who will use the materials in this book.

And last, but certainly not least, we wish to thank our editor from Corwin Press, Allyson Sharp; her editorial assistant, Nadia Kashper; our production editors, Beth Bernstein and Laureen Shea; and Corwin's art director, Anthony Paular, for answering our many e-mails, both in panic mode and not, for their immediate and efficient assistance.

Corwin Press gratefully acknowledges the contributions of the following reviewers:

Roberta Agar-Jacobsen
Teacher of the Deaf
Tacoma Public Schools
Tacoma, WA

Mary V. Compton
Associate Professor
Department of Specialized Education Services, Education of Deaf Children
The University of North Carolina at Greensboro
Greensboro, NC

Kenneth Morseon
Superintendent
Cleary School for the Deaf
Nesconset, NY

Sara Lynne Murrell
Instructional Coach
Elementary School
Simpsonville, SC

Sherilyn Renner
Teacher of the Deaf, Hard of Hearing
Bozeman Public Schools
Bozeman, MT

About the Authors

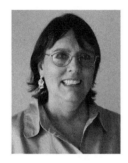

Susan R. Easterbrooks, EdD, is a Professor of Deaf Education in the Educational Psychology and Special Education Department in the College of Education at Georgia State University (http://education.gsu.edu/epse) and has been active in the field of deaf education for over 30 years. Dr. Easterbrooks has been a teacher, clinician, administrator, school psychologist, lecturer, and consultant and has authored numerous articles, chapters, and books on the education of children who are deaf and hard of hearing. She has participated actively on various local, state, and national committees. She currently serves as chair of the committee revising *Knowledge and Skills Needed by Teachers of the Deaf and Hard of Hearing* for the *Division for Communicative Disabilities and Deafness* of the *Council for Exceptional Children.* She participated in the development and revision of guidelines for services to students with hearing loss, published by the *National Association of State Directors of Special Education* and on the Special Needs committee of the *National Board for Professional Teaching Standards.* Dr. Easterbrooks resides in Gainesville, Georgia, with her husband and son.

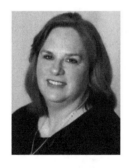

Ellen L. Estes is the Coordinator of the Katherine Hamm Center, an auditory-oral program for children with hearing losses at the Atlanta Speech School (www.atlantaspeech school.org). She has taught children with hearing losses for 30 years. She is a past-Chair of the International Professional Section of the Alexander Graham Bell Association for the Deaf and Hard of Hearing. She has written articles, conducted workshops, and advised schools throughout the country on many aspects of the language and literacy development of children who are deaf or hard of hearing. She resides in Powder Springs, Georgia, with her children and two very bad dogs.

Part 1

The Art of Intervention

Children who are deaf or hard of hearing face many challenges when learning to communicate. Communication difficulties can lead to problems with academic and social-emotional development. Helen Keller was once asked which was her greater challenge, her hearing loss, or her visual loss. She remarked that her hearing loss was more of a challenge because, while a vision loss separates one from things, a hearing loss separates one from people. We learn to communicate through our contact with others and through that communication we learn social and academic knowledge and skills.

Part 1 of this book consists of five chapters that are organized to reflect the developmental nature of children and the processes of listening to and using spoken language. For example, if you are working with a five-year-old child who is receiving services for the first time, it is appropriate for you to start with activities and skills associated with infants and toddlers. The science is the same for the newest learners; the art is in making early skills available through age-appropriate activities. As you read through these chapters, you may want to refer to Part 2: The Science of Intervention for more details about the reasons why you need to organize the environment in the ways we suggest. The chapters in Part 1 are as follows:

Chapter 1, "Listening and Spoken Language Interventions: A Model and Activities for Helping Children," identifies our *Model of Auditory, Speech, and Language Development*. In this chapter you will learn about the components of spoken communication you need to address and a format for thinking collectively about the components.

Chapter 2, "Early Detection and Intervention for Infants and Toddlers," discusses the approaches, practices, techniques, and strategies you will need to work with very young children with hearing loss.

Chapter 3, "Interventions for Preschoolers," presents the approaches, practices, techniques, and strategies needed for working with children who are developmentally in the three to six age range.

Chapter 4, "Interventions for Children in the Primary Grades," identifies the needs of young school attendees.

Chapter 5, "Developing Literacy Skills in Children With Hearing Losses," begins the discussion of how language and literacy are intertwined as well as the challenges that hearing loss imposes on literacy acquisition.

As a teacher in general or special education, your job is to (1) help children with hearing losses learn to communicate, and (2) help impart social and academic information while they learn to communicate. It's important you do this in supportive and creative ways. While the process is not always easy, it is always exciting.

Listening and Spoken Language Interventions 1

A Model and Activities for Helping Children

Children who can hear learn spoken language because they listen to it all the time. They listen to themselves and they listen to others. A child who is born with a hearing loss, however, must be taught to listen. We hear with our ears but we listen with our brains. A child who is deaf or hard of hearing must organize sounds in a way that makes sense.

The best way to help a child organize sounds is by relating them to language. Language is the master organizer of our world of thoughts, ideas, words, and sounds. The primary objective of this chapter is to provide a model that general and special education teachers may use to organize the components of listening to spoken language so that children will learn to understand and use them. This *Model of Auditory, Speech, and Language Development* is presented in detail in this chapter.

Spoken language is learned most easily through listening. In past years the concept of "learning to listen" to spoken language was called *auditory training* (Erber, 1982). This has been replaced by other designations such as *auditory brain development,* the term we use in this book, or *auditory perceptual development.* However you label it, learning to listen to language is a process best begun at birth and conducted over many years. During the process of learning to listen, children must perceive differences in spoken language that range from very large differences to very small. For example, a car horn is very different from a brother's laugh. The more experience a child has with listening, the smaller the differences in language he will be able to hear. A more experienced listener will hear the difference between "wipe your feet" and "go to sleep." These patterns are far too similar for new language listeners to differentiate.

A large part of learning to listen to language is the development of the *auditory feedback loop.* Children need to learn to listen to themselves and how they talk so that they can monitor their spoken language. The auditory feedback loop is a necessary precursor to babbling and supports all future spoken language development. See Chapter 6 for an in-depth explanation of the auditory feedback loop.

Teachers will see two different populations of young children with hearing loss. The first population needs intensive stimulation; the second population needs extensive remediation. A well-prepared, intensely stimulating environment can foster the natural emergence of listening and spoken language. This has been referred to as *facilitated language learning* (Desjardin, Eisenberg, & Hodapp, 2006) or *incidental language learning* (McConkey-Robbins, 1998), which follow patterns of normal development.

There are other deaf and hard of hearing children who are not able to master spoken language at typical rates due to reasons such as learning disorders, language deprivation, or a late start developing a visual language from poor models. These children need more direct instruction, or *didactic instruction,* which is more remedial in nature.

If you have a child who does not have a usable listening or language base in your classroom, you will need to become more didactic or direct in your instruction. Work very closely with a highly qualified teacher of the deaf. In this book, we assume that you are working with young children with hearing loss who are acquiring spoken language through listening.

LISTENING CHALLENGES THAT CHILDREN MUST OVERCOME

During auditory brain development, teachers must organize spoken language stimuli into discrete skills. We do this so that the message we ask the child to listen to is comprehensible to her brain. A child's hearing loss artificially creates a set of filters that we must consider when working with the child. Auditory brain development is the process of chipping away at these filters, which include:

- **Thinking about sounds.** The child must think about and then organize sounds. The process of organizing occurs by learning to detect, discriminate, identify, and comprehend what is heard (Erber, 1982). First, the child has to realize that sounds are there. Next, he has to know that one sound is different from another. After that, he learns that the sounds are associated with different objects or events. Finally, he needs to understand what the sounds mean. If a child's thinking filter can detect but not discriminate, you may say, for example, "See the bee," but she doesn't know if you said, "See the bee" or "See the tree."

- **Components of speech and language.** We have vowels and consonants; we have words and phrases; and we have strings of words that make up sentences. We can speak in a happy voice or a sad voice. Various parts of speech make up these features, along with prosody and intonation. If a child's language filter is only three words long and we say, "Time to take your bath. Get your rubber ducky and come here," the child's brain might hear only "bath ducky here." This may cause the child to think you want her to give her ducky a bath.

- **The world outside of the child.** There is an interaction between what is happening in the child's head and what is happening in the external world that he can see and touch. The more closely auditory information matches what is happening in the real world, the easier it will be for the child to acquire spoken language. For example, if the child is trying to hear the difference between "banana" and "apple," you wouldn't put a pear in front of him. Similarly, if you were trying to teach him to perceive the subtle difference between "a tree" and "a bee," you would not have the radio playing in the background.

- **Child actions.** Babies are capable of certain actions, while toddlers have a greater repertoire. Preschoolers have an even larger set of behaviors they can evoke with the school-age child the most sophisticated of all. It would not be appropriate to ask a school-age child to stop sucking on a bottle when she hears a sound. Conversely, you would not expect a three-month-old baby to draw a circle around a word. The actions we observe that tell us what a child can hear must match what she is developmentally able to do.

Awareness of the Whole Child

Teachers must consider all the needs of the whole child who is putting this listening and language puzzle together. This child has emotions. If he is unhappy, he won't care about your instruction. If he is sick, he may not have the energy to listen. If he is visually impaired, he may not be able to see or manipulate materials. If the home and school languages differ, he may be overwhelmed. The child also brings a whole set of world experiences to the language learning task. Some children have had lots of experiences, while others have not had as many. The more experiences a child has, the larger a base we can draw upon when teaching him to communicate.

Here's a pop quiz. Pick the label (letter) that best goes with the description (number).

Box 1.1   Pop Quiz

Match the numbers to the letters.	
1. Pointing to a picture	a. Thinking about sounds
2. The "p" sound in the word "pat"	b. The world outside the child
3. A box of beanie babies	c. Components of speech and language
4. Noticing that "ball" and "jump" sound different	d. Child actions

If you chose the following, you were correct: 1d, 2c, 3b, 4a. In the remainder of this chapter you will learn in greater detail about each of the four areas we consider when providing intervention.

MODEL OF AUDITORY, SPEECH, AND LANGUAGE DEVELOPMENT

We designed the *Model of Auditory, Speech, and Language Development* presented in this chapter to assist teachers in thinking about the many parts of speech, language, and listening that they must manage during spoken language instruction. The *Model of Auditory, Speech, and Language Development* (Figure 1.1) tells us that the brain (brain tasks) processes meaningful speech and language (listening and speaking skills) in a variety of contexts (external intervening factors and child actions). For example, we might have an objective that looks like this: *Marius will demonstrate discrimination (brain task) between the vowel sounds -oo- and -oa- (listening and speaking skill) when given a closed set of three objects such as a boot, a toy boat, and a toy bear (external factor, in this case, size of set) by pointing to the correct picture (child action).* In this lesson the teacher might show Marius three toys (boot, boat, bear), saying one of the three words (e.g., boat). We would then hope to see Marius pointing to the toy the teacher said.

Here's another example: *Marissa will demonstrate comprehension (brain task) of two-syllable –ing words (listening and speaking skill) said by the teacher when given a picture containing the word (external factor, in this case, contextual cues) by saying (child action) the word that the teacher is describing.* In this lesson we would see the teacher giving Marissa a picture of a lake scene with maybe a boat and kids swimming near the shore. The teacher would say, for example, "Listen. Someone is <u>moving</u> through the water. His arms are <u>turning</u>. He is <u>kicking.</u> What is he <u>doing</u>?" Our expectation is for Marissa to say, "Swimming." Figure 1.1 demonstrates how three of these components (brain task, listening or speaking skill, and external factors) come together for a good lesson plan.

The *Model of Auditory, Speech, and Language Development* provides a structure for determining appropriate objectives. Think of the brain tasks as progressing from the front of the model to the back of the model in terms of difficulty (first we detect; then we discriminate; then we identify; then we comprehend). Think of listening and speaking skills as instructional targets that progress from the left side of the model to the right in difficulty. First we notice suprasegmental patterns, followed by vowels, then consonants, and then connected speech. But that's not the whole story. As we move a skill along the levels, each level develops simultaneously in the child's listening repertoire. The external factors, shown on the right side of the cube, are situation specific. In addition, there are always child behavioral tasks involved in every lesson that are not reflected on the model. When setting a goal, think of the following pattern:

> *The child will demonstrate (brain task) a (listening and speaking skill) when (external factor) by (child action).*

Figure 1.1   *Model of Auditory, Speech, and Language Development*

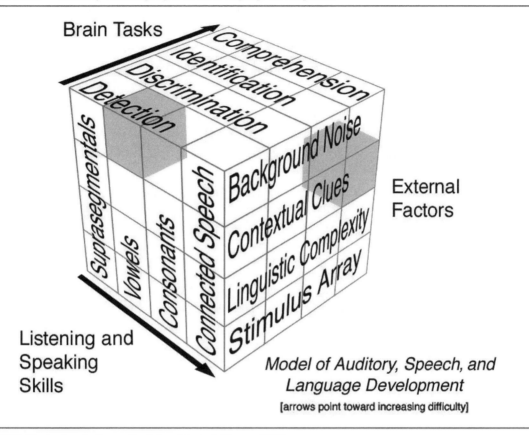

SOURCE: Illustration by James Poulakos, Mustafa Elsawy 2005.

Imagine now that you can pick out individual blocks from the three-dimensional model above. Locate the darkened block on the front face of the model. This might be telling us that Shantia will demonstrate that she detects (brain process) the vowels -a- and -oo- (listening and speaking skill) when associated with specific toys in the classroom such as "aaaaaa" for airplane and "oooo" for fire truck (external factors of context and background noise) by placing a ring on a spire (child's behavior or action). This is the sequence you will always follow in describing your objectives. See if you can come up with an example objective for the second block embedded in the back face of the model.

Parameter 1: Brain Tasks

Brain tasks tell us how a child's brain responds to sounds. Listening requires the child to think about what he hears; it is a thinking skill. In order to teach a child to listen, we must first understand what we expect him to think; that is, what we expect his mind to do with the information. There are four brain tasks: detection, discrimination, identification, and comprehension. The whole goal of auditory training is to teach the child to comprehend, or understand, information that he hears. Each of the different components of listening contributes to the development of comprehension. Activities must be meaningful and have sufficient content to make them useful to the child. Brain task development does not occur in a locked-step fashion. While you are helping the child comprehend (understand the meaning of) at one level (e.g., phrases of different length), you may also be helping him discriminate (detect the difference) at a different level (e.g., words with the same vowel).

Detection

> ⚜ **Essential Question #1**
>
> *Does the child hear the sound? Can he detect both the presence and absence of a sound? Does he demonstrate a response to a stimulus? Can he detect a range of sounds? Have you established a conditioned play response? Is there evidence of a spontaneous alerting response?*

The first component, or parameter, of brain tasks is *detection;* that is, the ability to respond to the presence of a sound or not to respond when there is no sound. We need to establish responding and nonresponding very quickly during auditory development. The child must learn to wait to respond to a sound; otherwise you may not be able to determine whether the child is actually hearing something or is just guessing. Children who do not have this response will wait for a certain amount of time to respond to a stimulus, but eventually they will not be able to wait any longer and will perform the expected behavior. If they are really listening for a sound, however, they will wait until they hear the stimulus before engaging in the behavior at hand. Waiting is not a problem if they truly are listening.

When developing this response to sound, you must focus first on the sounds that you expect the child can hear based on his aided audiogram. As explained in Chapter 6, an aided audiogram is a picture of a child's hearing response when he is wearing his hearing aid or cochlear implant. It is important to start auditory brain development with sounds we know the child can hear. For children over age one, you will teach a "conditioned play response"; that is, to react (e.g., throw a bean bag, stack a block) upon hearing a sound. You will also stimulate the development of spontaneous alerting responses that indicate that the child has heard the sound even when not specifically cued to listen. For example, when the child hears a sound, she may stop what she is doing and look for a sound, or she may vocalize, indicating that she has heard something. To develop the spontaneous response, have a third person in the room make a sound. Call the child's attention to the sound by describing the sound (e.g., "Oh look. She has a toy cow that says, 'moo.' I heard that moo. Did you?"). All children must have the ability to spontaneously alert to sound before you can begin working on any other level.

> **Example of a detection activity:** *Victoria will demonstrate detection (brain task) of the presence of various vowel sounds (listening and speaking skill) when the teacher provides a familiar stimulus (external factors) by dropping a block in a bucket (child action).*

Figure 1.2 Child Demonstrates Sound Detection by Placing a Ring on a Spire

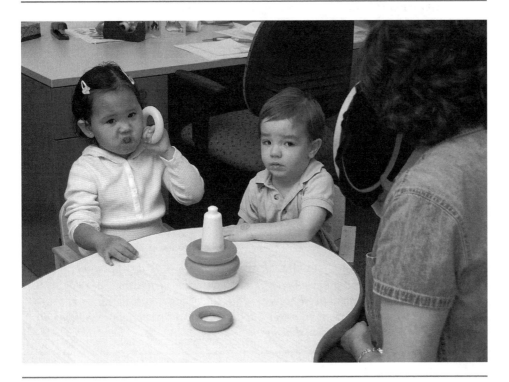

SOURCE: Photographed by John Zimmermann.

Discrimination

> ⚜ **Essential Question #2**
>
> *Discrimination is mostly used as a remedial tool for speech perception activities. But before we can do this, we need to answer several questions. Does the child indicate in some way that he knows that two sounds are the same or different? Does he indicate that he is listening for differences among sounds? Can he respond differently to different sounds?*

Once a child is able to detect speech, we move that skill along to the next brain task level. There, we ask the brain to tell the difference between or among sounds. This is called *auditory discrimination*. Auditory discrimination is defined as "the ability to perceive similarities and differences between and among sounds, to listen for differences among sounds, and to respond differently to different sounds" (Erber, 1982, p. 41). We want to determine if the child can tell that two sounds are different and if so, can he respond to these sounds in different ways. For example, "cow" versus "elephant" is a pattern that compares one syllable versus three syllables. At this level we might only be interested in whether or not he can tell that "elephant" is a longer word than "cow." If the child imitates an elephant's trunk movement when you say, "elephant" and a cow mooing when you say, "cow," then we know he can tell there is a difference in syllable length in these two sounds. The child may not know quite yet what the words are, but that comes next. For now, we are satisfied in knowing that the child can indicate to us in some way when he hears that the words are of different lengths.

It's important to note here that we move rapidly out of this brain task and into the task of identification, because auditory development activities are best conducted when sounds are meaningful to the child. Often we use this level of discrimination as a remedial tool. For example, when the child makes a speech error such as "tat" for "cat," you might say, "Listen, you said 'tat.' I said 'cat.' Can you hear the difference?" The purpose of using discrimination as a tool is for the child to compare two signals: a correct one and an incorrect one. This is the beginning of what is called "auditory self-monitoring" or "auditory feedback" which involves learning to modify one's own speech based on what one hears. For very young children who are just learning to listen, however, discrimination in its most basic forms may be actual objectives.

> **Example of a discrimination activity:** *Ahmed will demonstrate discrimination (brain task) between words with and without a final-s/z ending (listening and speaking skill) such as cat/cats, dog/dogs, tree/trees when the teacher says cat/cat versus cat/cats (external factor) by holding up his finger if the words are different and not holding up a finger if they are the same (child action).*

Figure 1.3   Child Discriminates Words With and Without Final-s Endings

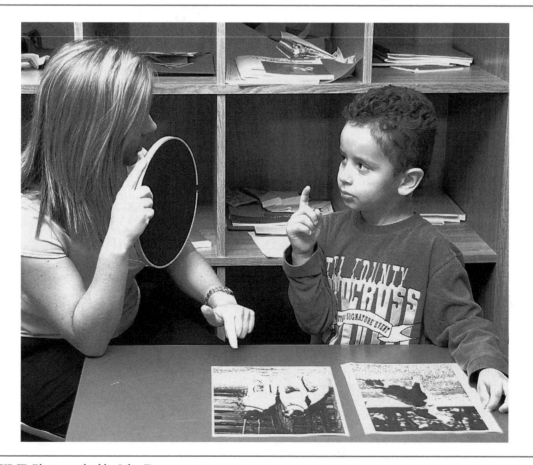

Identification

> ⚜ **Essential Question #3**
>
> *Can the child understand labels associated with a speech stimulus by copying what was said or pointing to an object, picture or word?*

Once the child is able to discriminate sounds, we begin to help her attach meaning to the sounds. We accomplish this through identification activities. Another word for identification is *recognition*. The child recognizes an acoustic pattern as the label for a specific object, event, person, or action. The goal is for the child either to repeat what she heard or to point to a picture or a printed word that represents the stimulus. Here's an example: You may be working with a child on a task where she is shown three objects, each of which represents a particular sound. Our objective is for her to identify the correct object or repeat the stimulus (e.g., jump, shhh, or beep-beep-beep) when she hears the teacher produce the sound. This is called auditory identification or auditory association.

> **Example of an identification activity:** *Maisha will demonstrate identification (brain task) of words of differing length (listening and speaking skill) when given a choice of three objects (external factor) by imitating speech or selecting the object (child action) that goes with stimulus presented, such as a boy, a baby, and grandfather.*

Comprehension

> ⚜ **Essential Question #4**
>
> *Can the child make higher-level associations between sounds and events or objects? Does he understand the meaning of what you are saying? Can he answer questions appropriately? Can he follow directions?*

Comprehension is the primary goal of listening instruction. Our whole focus is to make sure the child understands what he hears. Comprehension occurs when the child demonstrates the ability to understand the meaning of speech and when his response is quantitatively different from the stimulus presented. Another word for comprehension is *understanding*. Because comprehension is a process, we write comprehension goals differently from other goals. We must depend on the child's responses to demonstrate comprehension.

Another word we can associate with comprehension is *reformulation*. When doing a comprehension activity, we ask the child to listen and then to reformulate the information is some way that lets us know he understands it. The child will demonstrate comprehension by doing some action or changing the task around in a quantitatively measurable or visible way. This action will become the objective of your lesson. In other words, we know that the child understands what we have said because he *does* something appropriately related to the stimulus. For example, if you say, "Wash your hands" versus "Sit down," we can assume the child comprehends what we said if she does the correct task.

Following directions and answering questions appropriately are two good ways of showing that comprehension has occurred. You are looking for some indication that the child has derived meaning from what you have said. You want to know not only that she can hear the stimulus but also that she can understand the language or meaning of the stimulus.

Auditory comprehension is composed of the following four components: auditory memory, following one-step commands with one critical element, auditory sequencing, and auditory integration. *Auditory memory* is demonstrated when the child remembers what she has heard (e.g., teacher reads a story, child acts out the story). *Following one-step commands with one critical element* involves using one word to instruct the child to act out something in a story or game such as "jump" or "push." Once the child can act out one-word instructions our next objective is *auditory sequencing*, where the child must remember things in order, such as two-step commands or two actions in a story, building eventually to three and four commands or actions. The final comprehension skill involves *auditory integration*, where the child must think about the language she has heard for the purpose of integrating language and thinking. For example, we might ask, "What color do you get when you mix blue and yellow?" This is by far the most difficult level of comprehension, but it is also the whole point of why we do auditory training. In order to reach this level, the child needs adequate perception of sound as well as knowledge of language. Without the ability to integrate listening, language, and thinking, the child will be at a disadvantage in developing spoken language and in being successful upon entering school.

Example of a comprehension activity: *Josette will answer "what" and "where" questions (child action) about a story (listening and speaking skill) that the teacher reads to her (external factor).*

Figure 1.4   Children Answer Questions About a Story

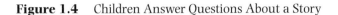

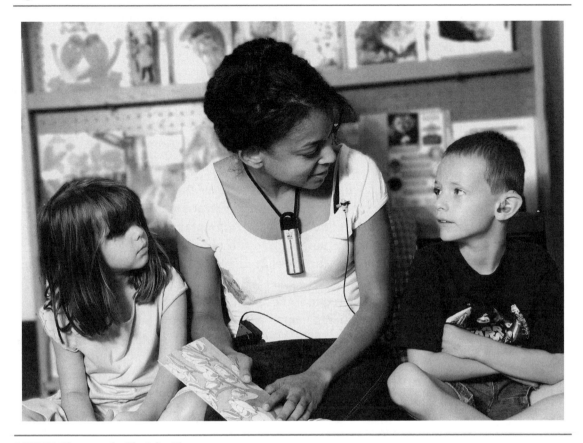

SOURCE: Photographed by John Zimmermann.

Remember, comprehension objectives are written differently from other brain task objectives because it is a process. Comprehension *is* the brain task, but it is measured by what the child produces. It involves actively *thinking with language* internally.

Parameter 2: Listening and Speaking Skills

Listening is the foundation of spoken language. If you want a child to learn to speak the language of his home and culture, then you must teach him to learn to listen to that language. We start with the brain tasks above, but the brain has to have some information to think about. The information we give a child's brain to think about in auditory training is meaningful, spoken language. Spoken language objectives (both the listening side of the coin and the speaking side of the coin) form the core of instructional units or targets and may be broken into categories. Remember, we artificially separate out spoken language skills so we can be sure that what we are asking the brain to think about is comprehensible; that is, it is in a small and meaningful enough unit that the brain will be able to pay attention to it.

The components of listening and speaking skills are suprasegmentals, vowels and diphthongs, words, phrases, and connected speech. They are the building blocks of spoken language, our main targets or objectives.

Suprasegmentals

✤ **Essential Question #5**

Does the child demonstrate that he hears the differences among patterns of sound that are composed of differing durational, stress, intonational, or phrasing elements?

The first and simplest level where children learn to perceive differences inherent in spoken language is the suprasegmental level. At the suprasegmental level we work on: pattern perception, duration patterns, stress (requiring duration and intensity pattern changes), intonation (requiring duration, intensity, and pitch pattern changes), and phrasing (requiring intonation pattern changes). See Chapter 6 for in-depth information on duration, intensity, and pitch.

Pattern perception requires the child to do something different based on the presentation of two different sound patterns. We may ask the child to listen to the difference between a long sound and a short sound or an intermittent sound and a prolonged sound. For example, we can use the stimulus "pull" versus the stimulus "throw the bean bag," where we might have the child pull some Pop-It beads or throw a bean bag based on which pattern he has heard. It is not necessary for the child to understand what "pull" means or what "throw the bean bag" means, only that he recognizes that one pattern goes with one action and the other pattern goes with another action. He can do the activity just by recognizing the pattern.

Perception of duration requires the child to listen to durational patterns beginning with simple patterns such as the one described above, and then moving into durational patterns associated with long versus short sounds such as "ruff" versus "meow." Even if the child can't hear the frequency changes she can still determine that one is short and one is longer. The objective isn't vowels per se, but vowel pattern duration. With older children, we return to working on duration in the form of syllable accent. The accent on syllables is not conveyed by loudness but by duration, so older children can work on listening to and saying words such as **pre**-sent and pre-**sent** or **con**-tent and con-**tent**.

Perception of stress refers to the accenting done across a sentence, such as "Put **that** there," referring to the object versus, "Put that **there**," referring to the location. In this instance the child would have to identify whether the stress caused the focus of the sentence to be on the object or on the location. Stress perception requires a combination of duration and intensity patterns. Listen to yourself as you say "that" and "there" in the examples above. You will notice that the words are not only louder but longer as well when they are the stressed word of the sentence.

Perception of intonation refers to the rise and fall of inflection within a sentence, such as the rising intonation of a yes/no question. Perception and production of intonation require duration, intensity, and pitch changes across a phrase. It includes activities that help the child listen to the entire speech envelope, or the intonational ebb and flow of a particular spoken utterance. For example, we would have different ebb and flow when we say, "George is Norm's best friend," if we meant it as truth versus if we meant it sarcastically.

Perception of phrasing requires the listener to understand that certain words go together, such as the phrase "in the car," which we actually run together quite rapidly in normal speech. Understanding and using phrasing is dependent upon good intonational perception and use. In the real world, when people speak to us or when we speak, we run words together. Think of the phrase "OK. I have got to go." In the real world we would phrase it in a pattern something like "nnn K, Iguttago." You can see why it would be difficult for a developing child to figure out this sentence if he had to pay attention to each word rather than to the entire pattern.

> **Example of a suprasegmental activity:** *Andy will demonstrate identification (brain task) of common two and three element intonation patterns (listening and speaking skill) associated with everyday experiences (external factor of context) when given three pictures (external factor of closed set) by pointing (child action) to the correct picture.*

Figure 1.5 Children Identify Spoken Language Patterns

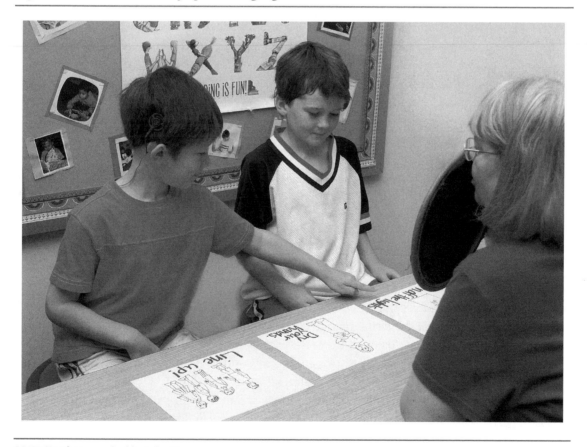

SOURCE: Photographed by John Zimmermann.

In this lesson the teacher has a folder of a dozen different captioned pictures taken of everyday experiences in the classroom. Examples are: Line up. Sit down. Time for lunch. Wash your hands. Turn off the lights, please. Push your chair to the table. The teacher sets out three pictures, being careful to pick phrases of three different lengths (e.g., Line up. Wash your hands. Turn off the lights, please.). She reads the captions under the picture to the child, and has him repeat them. Then, covering her mouth, she says the caption and asks Andy to point. Andy's correct response will earn him a puzzle piece, all of which he can put together at the end of the session.

Vowels and Consonants

⚜ Essential Question #6

When helping a child listen to the differences between vowels and consonants, do you provide a sufficiently noticeable difference by working between vowel or consonant categories before working within vowel or consonant categories?

Vowels and consonants are the *segmental sounds* of speech, as opposed to the suprasegmental sounds (i.e., intensity, duration, and pitch). Another word for a segmental sound is an *elemental* sound. Segmental aspects of speech are the frequency components of vowels or the manner, place, and voicing of consonants that differentiate one speech sound from another. See Chapter 6 for more information on the components of speech. When developing lesson activities, it is important to ensure the distinctions between the sounds are audible. It is easy to incorporate too many aspects of a sound, such as duration or intensity, into a lesson. Remember, we are artificially breaking down the sounds to make the differences apparent.

Also, we do not want to confuse the child by adding in suprasegmental information, such as making one vowel sound longer and the other shorter. If we did that, the child would probably respond to the difference in duration rather than the difference in the way the two vowels sounded. When working on any particular listening skill, it is always good practice to keep the stimuli constant and not add in too many confounding characteristics.

In determining whether a child can hear the differences between vowels, you must carefully review the child's audiograms. Find out as much information about the frequencies the child can hear. Look at the first and second formants of the vowels as they relate to the audiologic information you have about the child to determine how much of the sound the child can hear. See Chapter 6 for more information on formants and audiograms.

The vowels listed on Table 1.1 are arranged from easiest to hear to hardest to differentiate. The easiest sounds to hear are the diphthongs because of the transition that occurs when saying them. The next easiest sounds are the Group 1 sounds because the second formants of these sounds fall in the lower frequencies. The Group 2 vowels are more difficult to hear because they have a mid-frequency second formant. The Group 3 vowels—where the second formants fall in the higher frequency ranges—are the most difficult to hear. Say these groupings to yourself and you should be able to detect both changes in frequency and changes in tongue location.

When you begin helping students, listen to the difference between vowels. Start with a diphthong, and compare it to a Group 3 sound because the differences are more noticeable. Listen to yourself say "i-e" as in *pie* and "a-e" as in *pay,* repeatedly alternating the two as in "i-e, a-e, i-e, a-e." Now listen to yourself say, "i-e" as in *eye* and "-i-" as in *pin* repeatedly as in "i-e, -i-, i-e, -i-." Which pair sounds and feels most different? Yes, the second set. This is the kind of contrast we want to present to the child.

Always work on contrasts between groups before you begin to work on contrasts within groups because all of the sounds within a group have similar second formants and will sound similar to the child with a hearing loss. You want the child to have successful listening experiences before giving him the challenging experiences. Between-group comparisons are much easier to make than within-group comparisons.

Table 1.1   Frequency Information for Vowels

Level of Difference	Category
F2 (available) ↓ F2 (difficult to hear)	Diphthongs: i-e, a-e, oa, ou, u-e, oi Group 1 vowels: aw, -oo-, oo Group 2 vowels: -o-, -u-. er Group 3 vowels: ee. -a-. -i-. -e-

SOURCES: Biedenstein, Davidson, and Moog (1995); Denes and Pinson (1993); Erber (1982); Ling and Ling (1978).

When helping a child learn to listen to consonants, you must consider their relative frequency (Hz) patterns. Table 1.2 presents groups of consonants that range from the lowest frequencies to the highest frequencies. Although nasal sounds are the lowest in frequency, they are also very soft sounds and can be difficult for the child to hear. Be sure to take extra care in providing sufficient loudness to the child when working on the lowest frequency sounds. Regarding high-frequency sounds, children with cochlear implants will be able to hear those sounds (assuming their devices are optimally set); however, some children with hearing aids may not have sufficient hearing to bring these higher sounds into an accessible range. Again, remember to look at a child's audiogram relative to the frequency characteristics of a sound to understand how best to proceed. As with the vowels, always have the child listen to between-group contrasts before listening to within-group contrasts. See Chapter 6 for more information on these concepts.

When working on vowels and consonants, it's important to take into consideration that some speech sounds are loud and some are quiet. Sometimes strong sounds can mask or overpower weaker sounds. You may be able to compensate for this by increasing the intensity of the weaker sound. If you cannot do this, then you will probably need to choose a different contrast for developing the sound. See Chapter 6 for information on intensity of sounds.

Table 1.2   Frequency Information for Consonants

Frequency Level	Consonants
Low-frequency consonants	m, b, d, n, -ng
High-frequency consonants	voiceless th, s, f, k, g, h, p, t, sh, ch
Mid-frequency consonants	r, l
Consonants with low- and high-frequency components	z, zh, v, voiced th, j

SOURCE: From *The Speech Chain: The Physics and Biology of Spoken Language* by Peter B. Denes and Elliott N. Pinson, copyright © 1993 by W. H. Freeman and Company. Reprinted by permission of Henry Holt and Company, LLC.

> **Example #1 of a segmental activity:** *Steven will demonstrate identification (brain task) of minimal pairs of voiced and voiceless plosives (listening and speaking skill) when given a choice of two words (external factor of closed set) by pointing to the correct word (child action).*

In this activity, we would see the teacher write pairs of words such as pear/bear or pig/big for Steven to see. The teacher says all the words to Steven and has him attempt to say them back, working on getting the words into his personal feedback system. Finally, the teacher says one of the words in the pair, and Steven points to the word she said (see Figure 1.6).

Figure 1.6   Child Discriminates Between Words Starting With /b/ or /p/

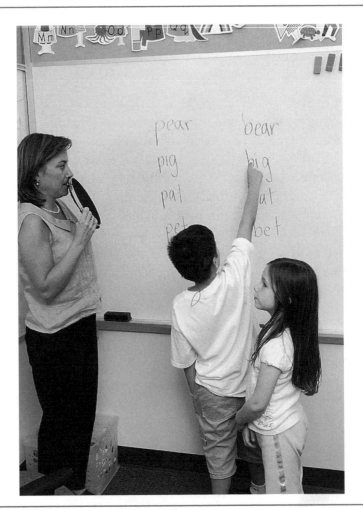

SOURCE: Photographed by John Zimmermann.

Example #2 of a segmental activity: *Ariel will demonstrate identification (brain task) of the long vowels i-e and o-e (listening and speaking skill) in single syllable words (external factor of context) when shown three objects (external factor of size of set) by picking the correct object and repeating the word (child action).*

In this lesson the teacher uses toys representing words that have diphthong sounds in them. Sample objects are plastic replicas of a fly, a pie, a rake, a cake, a boat, and a rope. The teacher pulls the toys from a box, goes over the words with the student, and verifies that she understands what to do with each object (such as eat the pie or rake leaves). The teacher sets out one object corresponding to each diphthong in a set of three and then says, "Give me the _____." If Ariel gives her the correct object, she gets to pretend to be the teacher on the next turn.

Connected Speech

⚜ Essential Question #7

Can the child identify critical elements in connected discourse? Can she identify elements in practiced sentences, in conversation, and in connected discourse tracking?

The final level of speech perception where you will do specific auditory development activities is the level of connected speech, or spoken language per se. This is where your language and speech goals will merge most obviously. Connected speech includes words, phrases, sentences, and longer discourse.

Once the child is able to hear the differences among various suprasegmental patterns, and when he has developed a listening repertoire of vowels and consonants in words, we ask him to respond to phrases and sentences. We begin by limiting the number of critical elements he must address. For example, we have the child listen for two critical elements (blue shoe versus red sock) before we have the child listen for three critical elements (big yellow star versus little green heart). A second form of connected speech (i.e., connected language) that we have the child listen to is *practiced* sentences. Examples include songs or poems or very short stories that we have written on chart paper. Although the sentence may include a number of elements, we might ask the child to focus only on a particular phrase or word grouping. For example, we might ask him to recall the last few words of a line of a poem, or we might ask him to remember "fee, fi, fo, fum" when listening to the story of *Jack and the*

Beanstalk. After the child is able to hear messages in practiced sentences, we might ask him to engage in spontaneous conversations where we provide the topic. Finally, we will ask the child to tell us what we said when we have not provided the topic of the conversation.

Connected discourse tracking is a specific teaching strategy that uses storybooks that are on a language level appropriate for the students. At the first level, the teacher reads the story and then asks the child to describe what occurred in the story. At the next level the teacher asks the children to follow along in their books, pointing to the words as they are read. At the highest level of difficulty, the teacher would read a phrase or sentence, then pause and have the child repeat exactly what he heard. This technique can be used to carry over important language goals or speech targets.

> **Example of a connected speech-language activity:** *Cody will demonstrate identification (brain task) of the targeted connected-speech phrases "in a box/tree/car" and so on (listening and speaking skill) from the book* Green Eggs and Ham *(external factor of closed set) when read by the teacher in a quiet room and one-to-one interaction (external factor of minimal background noise) by completing the target speech phrase (child action).*

In this lesson, Cody and his teacher will have read and discussed the story several times prior to this experience. They will have developed picture charts that represent the concepts "in a house," "in a box," "in a car," "in a tree," "in the dark," and "in the rain." In this lesson the teacher reads the story, and then Cody points to the picture and repeats the phrase when the teacher reads the target phrase.

Speech Perception Categories

A good way to determine the level of perception to begin your listening activities is to use the results of speech perception testing conducted by the audiologist and the results of tests such as the *Early Speech Perception Test* (ESP; Moog & Geers, 1990). These tests help to place children into one of six categories (see Table 1.3). They will give you information both about what the child can do successfully and what you need to focus on as a target or objective.

Perception of connected speech and language is only one side of the coin. We must also carefully examine the normal developmental stages and phases of language itself. Language develops sequentially in the following manner: preverbal communication, preinflected communication, simple sentences, compound sentences, complex sentences, and finally compound-complex sentences.

Parameter 3: External Factors

It is important to carefully control any external factors surrounding the lesson that make it more or less challenging. Note in the model (Figure 1.1) that there is no arrow on this parameter. This is because external factors do not

Table 1.3   Speech Perception Categories

Category	Characteristic
0	No detection of speech
1	Detection
2	Pattern perception
3	Beginning word identification
4	Word identification through vowel recognition
5	Word identification through consonant recognition
6	Open-set word recognition

SOURCES: Cheng, Grant, and Niparko (1999); Geers (1994); Moog and Geers (1990); Staller, Beiter, Brimacombe, Mecklenburg, and Arndt (1991).

occur along a continuum but rather all four are present in some way during any classroom listening task. Many categories of external factors exist that can influence a lesson. The child's current health status is another factor addressed earlier in the chapter but not identified in our model. Illnesses, middle ear problems, and other physical factors will affect the child's ability to perform a task. In this model we have identified only those factors over which the teacher has control that commonly influence the environment in which the lesson is being conducted and the materials being used. It is important that you understand the unique nature of the child with whom you are working so that you may account for other external factors not mentioned here.

In general there are four broad categories of external factors: the background or physical environment in which the lesson is being conducted; the linguistic environment in which the listening or speaking skill is couched; the contextual environment associated with the materials used and actions of the teacher; and the stimulus array. All of these provide the framework that you will establish before you ask the child to apply a brain task to an intended listening and speaking skill. While you work on the different levels of perception and the different skill levels, you also manipulate the context in which a task is set. Listening becomes harder as you increase the brain task and type of skill. It is also harder when the environment, materials, and teacher actions are manipulated as well. When you work on a new skill or a new level, you need to back off on the difficulty of the other components to keep the listening challenge within the child's grasp. For example, if the child is just beginning to listen to the difference between a pattern of three elements and a pattern of two elements, then you would want to have a closed set of options from which to choose rather than leaving the choices open-ended. Tasks should be challenging but not out of reach; comprehensible, but not confusing.

Stimulus Array

⚜ Essential Question #8

Is the child able to respond to an open-set stimulus array, or does he need a closed or a limited set? Does the child need to have materials modified?

One component of the environment you want to control is the *stimulus array,* that is, the material that is sitting in front of the child. We can modify this stimulus by controlling the size of the set. Sets of materials can be open or closed. A *closed set* has a specified number of responses from which to choose. The student is aware that you will say something that relates to one of the pictures or manipulatable objects in front of him or a specific topic under discussion (e.g., zoo animals). For example, if you want the child to listen to one and three syllable differences, you might use the names of students in the class. The child is already familiar with these names and the number of choices is limited. You might say, "Sam" versus "Anthony." Here, the child is not overly challenged because only a small number of possibilities exist. You can increase and decrease the size of the set to change the level of difficulty of the listening task.

In a *limited set,* the child has natural, situational, or contextual cues that define the set but you have not actually told him what the possible answers are, as is the case with a closed set. For example, when reading a book with a cow and sheep, the child can probably figure out that you aren't going to say the word "football." Another example would be a task where all the pictures represent "ch" words but the child does not know the sentence within which you are going to put the word. He has a frame of reference for what you are going to say but does not know the exact words you will choose.

In an *open set* the situational and contextual cues are minimal. The child has no cues as to what you are going to say. When you are doing open-set tasks you can switch topics a lot. For example, you might talk about one topic for two or three conversational turns but then would switch the topic so that the child must be on his toes to listen for what you are saying.

Another way we manipulate the stimulus array is by type of object. Objects can be real (real peaches), three-dimensional (plastic peaches), pictorial (pictures of peaches or drawings of peaches), or representational (as in the spoken word, "peach," or the written word, **peach**). When children are very new to the listening experience or are very young, they benefit from materials that are more real than virtual or representational.

We can also modify the materials we are using by adapting them in some fashion. Color-coding, making material tactile, categorizing, classifying, reorganizing, graphing, charting, and writing are only some of the ways that teachers manipulate materials to enhance the concepts they are trying to help young children grasp.

> **Example of a size of set activity:** *Cara will demonstrate discrimination (brain task) between two-syllable and three-syllable phrase patterns (listening and speaking skill) when given a closed set of two items in the stimulus array (external factor) by pointing to two or three blocks (child action).*

In this lesson the teacher chooses two- and three-syllable words or phrases with which Cara has had experience. These include the names of stores that she is familiar with such as Target, Wal-Mart, Dairy Queen, or Pizza Hut. The teacher sets two blocks to Cara's left and three blocks to Cara's right. She shows pictures of the stores and helps Cara count out the number of syllables in their names using the blocks. After doing this for all the store names, the teacher sets out one picture of a two-syllable store name and one of a three-syllable store name. She instructs Cara to push the set of two blocks toward her if the name has two syllables and to push the set of three blocks toward her if the name has three syllables. Next, the teacher takes out two pictures (one with a two-syllable phrase and the other with a three-syllable phrase), covers her mouth with a screen, and says one of the store names. Cara points to the picture and pushes the correct pile of blocks to the teacher and the teacher replaces the blocks. The teacher replaces the picture with another having the same number of syllables. The size of the set is kept at two choices. After the lesson is over, Cara plays with her pile of blocks.

Linguistic Complexity

> ### ⚜ Essential Question #9
>
> *At what linguistic level is this child? What are the key traits of that linguistic level? In what basic level of complexity must I place stimuli: single words or phrases? Can my child respond to stimuli in carrier phrases, and where within the phrase should the stimulus reside? How many elements can the child retain?*

Another external factor you must address is the complexity of the language in which you place the stimulus. The easiest level is the single-word level. To make a task a little more challenging, the teacher uses a carrier phrase and asks the student to identify the word at the end of the phrase or sentence. An example would be: "Find the car, find the shoe, or, give me the car, give me the shoe." A more difficult level contains the word in the middle of the sentence such as, "Put the cow in the barn. Put the horse in the barn." In these levels, the child has to listen for only one critical element; that is, the carrier phrase remains the same and the stimulus word is the only thing that changes.

In the next higher level, we increase the number of critical elements the child must listen to, such as "Put the <u>cow/horse/sheep</u> **(1)** in the <u>wagon/field/barn</u> **(2)**," so that two critical elements change. After the child masters this, the teacher increases the difficulty by making three things changeable—for example, "Put the <u>brown/black/white</u> **(1)** <u>cow/horse/sheep</u> **(2)** in the <u>wagon/field/barn</u> **(3)**"—then four—for example, "Put the <u>big/little</u> **(1)** <u>brown/black/white</u> **(2)** <u>cow/horse/sheep</u> **(3)** in the <u>wagon/field/barn</u> **(4)**"—then more. As the number of elements increases, so does the grammatical difficulty. It is important that you become familiar with the grammatical aspects associated with the major stages of grammar: preinflected phrases (e.g., Daddy go bye-bye?), simple sentences, compound sentences, complex sentences, and compound-complex sentences. If your child is not able to understand simple sentences, then do not place a stimulus word within a compound sentence.

> **Example of a linguistic complexity activity (two critical elements):** *Destiny will demonstrate comprehension (brain task) of the meaning of "in" and "on" and a noun (listening and speaking skill) when the teacher identifies locations within the phrase "the ____" (external factor) by placing an object in that location (child action).*

In this lesson we see Destiny and her teacher playing with a Press-and-Peel farm set. The teacher hands Destiny a farm animal piece such as a chicken and makes sure that Destiny knows the locations ("Show me the barn; the house; the coop"). Covering her mouth with a screened hoop, she tells Destiny to put the chicken "in the barn." Destiny responds appropriately by sticking the chicken to the barn. As a reward, the teacher lets her choose the next farm animal, and they continue the game.

Contextual Cues

> ❧ **Essential Question #10**
>
> *Does the child need a lot of verbal, visual, pictorial, or situational cues, or does she understand auditory tasks within minimal context?*

Another area that you can manipulate to make a task harder or easier is the amount of contextual cues you give. For example, you might start by saying that you are going to talk about the girls in the class. You would follow this by saying, "Sally has a pretty red bow in her hair," and ask the child to repeat what he heard, or you might have a less specific context such as, "Now we are going to talk about people in school." You would still talk about Sally and her bow, but you have given a less specific context to the child. You can also take advantage of situational cues. For example, if it is recess time and everyone is getting ready to go out, you might ask the child to listen to and repeat, "Put your coat on." The child would know from the context that you aren't going to say, "Go brush your teeth." Finally, you can use storybooks or pictures as stimuli for listening. These would give the child the context so that if you were looking at a picture of children on a playground, he could predict that you wouldn't say something like, "My aunt got a new red car."

> **Example of a contextual cues activity:** *Armel will state (child action implying the brain task of comprehension) the name of an object in a category (listening and speaking skill) when the teacher gives a category such as fruit or toys (external factor of open set).*

Note that the category is a limited set (e.g., category names: fruit, animals, toys, etc.), but Armel must generate an answer. Armel and his class have been studying categories of things around the house. In this activity the teacher has given each child a stack of cards with words such as apple, fish, ball, shirt on them. She covers her mouth and says, "Who has a fruit?" The child with a fruit shows his card and names it (e.g., apple).

Background Noise

> ⚜ Essential Question #11
>
> *Is the child able to listen in all levels of noise from quiet to competing messages?*

We live in a noisy world, and children need to learn to listen within the context of noise. When a child is first listening, however, we need to make sure that there are no external distractions. If the child is not able to ignore sounds in the environment, you may want to do some initial listening activities in a quiet room. Once the child has achieved a listening goal in quiet, then you can make your lessons a little more challenging by increasing the competing noise. Noise levels are described as quiet (no other sounds), soft ambient noise (a sound-treated room with other activities occurring), normal ambient noise (a regular room with other students in it), loud ambient noise (a room with loud equipment such as an air conditioner in it, or near the gymnasium), and competing noise (such as the cafeteria). To make an activity easier, check to see that you are not competing for the child's attention with distracting noise in the room. Children live and play in a big world outside of the therapy room or classroom. To make any task harder, increase the amount and type of ambient noise. You can make any of the activities described above harder by turning a radio on softly in the background, or by doing the activity in a different location.

Parameter 4: Child Actions

> ⚜ Essential Question #12
>
> *Are the activities you are asking the child to do age and interest appropriate?*

One parameter that our model does not depict is the real child who is learning to listen. Whenever this child engages in speech and language tasks in various contexts of difficulty, he is not simply going to sit there passively. He is going to *do* something. Children, or all humans for that matter, have no choice but to engage in some kind of behavior. Therefore, be sure to ask the child to perform age-appropriate behavior.

Child behavioral tasks associated with each lesson are determined by the age, skill level, cognitive level, and physical challenges facing the child. For example, we would not expect a six-month-old to place plastic objects into appropriate categories. Nor would we ask a visually impaired child to look at two pictures and choose the correct one. This again is something that the teacher must take into consideration when designing an activity. Actions may include, but are by no means limited to pointing, showing, changing, drawing, making, moving, writing, saying, rearranging, dropping, throwing, pushing, jumping over, crawling under, standing beside, rolling, taking, sorting, and hundreds of other real actions. The more enticing the action, the more likely it is that you will maintain the child's interest in what you are doing. Listening is a skill that is used in every aspect of the human experience, not just when we are sitting at a table in front of the teacher. For this reason, make your activities and child actions as real and fun and meaningful as you can.

Finally, we come back full circle to the whole child. In addition to all the factors of spoken language development and all the factors associated with the development of a good lesson, remember, we are dealing with a real person. This little person may come from a home where English is not the spoken language. She may have additional disabilities that limit her ability to use her cognitive, sensory, or motor skills. She may have come to the listening and language learning task later than other children. She may be distractible, tired, hungry, sad, bored, temperamental, or confused. Her parents may differ in their ability to participate in the process. She may have siblings with other, greater needs, which take precedence over her communication development. Never forget that you are working with a special, unique individual.

SUMMARY

This chapter presents 12 sets of essential questions to help organize the parameters for spoken language intervention. The parameters include brain tasks, speech and language skills, external factors, and child actions. The sets of questions are:

1. Does the child hear the sound? Can he detect both the presence and absence of a sound? Does he demonstrate a response to a stimulus? Can he detect a range of sounds? Have you established a conditioned play response? Is there evidence of a spontaneous alerting response?

2. Discrimination is mostly used as a remedial tool for speech perception activities, but before we can do this, we need to answer several questions. Does the child indicate in some way that he knows two sounds are the same or different? Does he indicate that he is listening for differences among sounds? Can he respond differently to different sounds?

3. Can the child apply a label to a speech stimulus by copying what was said or pointing to an object, picture, or word?

4. Can the child make higher-level associations between sounds and events or objects? Does he understand the meaning of what you are saying? Can he answer questions appropriately? Can he follow directions?

5. Does the child demonstrate that he hears the differences among patterns of sound that are comprised of differing durational, stress, intonational, or phrasing elements?

6. When helping a child listen to the differences between vowels and consonants, are you providing a sufficiently noticeable difference by working between vowel or consonant categories before working within vowel or consonant categories?

7. Can the child identify critical elements in connected discourse? Can she identify elements in practiced sentences, in conversation, and in connected discourse tracking?

8. Is the child able to respond to an open-set stimulus array, or does he need a closed or a limited set? Does the child need to have materials modified?

9. At what linguistic level is this child? What are the key traits of that linguistic level? In what basic level of complexity must I place stimuli: single words or phrases? Can my child respond to stimuli in carrier phrases, and where within the phrase should the stimulus reside? How many elements can the child retain?

10. Does the child need a lot of verbal, visual, pictorial, or situational cues, or does she understand auditory tasks within minimal context?

11. Is the child able to listen in all levels of noise from quiet to competing messages?

12. Are the activities you are asking the child to do age and interest appropriate?

Keep these questions in mind as you read through the intervention chapters, which focus on planning and conducting appropriate activities to help children listen to and use spoken language.

Early Detection and Intervention for Infants and Toddlers 2

This chapter begins a four-chapter sequence of intervention, starting with babies and toddlers. In this chapter we describe the reasons why we do what we do to help the littlest children learn to communicate. We have four objectives in this chapter. First, we describe universal newborn hearing screening and early intervention. Next we explore services needed by infants and toddlers with hearing loss and their families. Then we discuss developmental issues that are going on at this stage, and finally we present developmentally appropriate interventions.

Babies are watchers and listeners; they are very little and don't do much yet. Although it may appear that they simply sit, watch, listen, flail and kick, and make noises, actually they are little "sensory sponges," taking in everything that comes within seeing, hearing, touching, tasting, or smelling range. An important strategy during these first years is to bring everything within close range of infants and toddlers to stimulate their senses in a way that will set the sensory sponge process into motion.

EARLY DETECTION AND INTERVENTION

Historically, an undetected hearing loss has had serious consequences. Many children with hearing loss have repeated grades in school or lagged behind their peers in communication and academics. However, recent technological advances, legal mandates, and new evidence regarding the consequences of early intervention have allowed us to make major advances in outcomes for children with hearing loss. Advances in technology have dramatically increased the ease and success with which hospitals can screen the hearing of newborns. Legal mandates, including Part C of the Individuals with Disabilities

Education Act of 1997 (now IDEA 2004), outline policies that states should follow to make sure that all newborns have their hearing tested. (The more recent version of the law aligns IDEA with the No Child Left Behind legislation. In addition, it specifically allows consideration of cued speech and American Sign Language in early intervention services.) Evidence supporting the success of early hearing screening (Mehl & Thomson, 2002) and the effectiveness of early intervention beginning in infancy (Calderon, 2000; Sass-Lehrer & Bodner-Johnson, 2003; Yoshinaga-Itano, Sedey, Coulter, & Mehl, 1998) is persuasive.

Today, most newborns are screened for potential hearing loss in the nursery. About three out of every 1,000 newborns have a hearing loss. Losses can range from mild to profound. The American Speech-Language-Hearing Association (ASHA) supports the goal of early intervention in all babies by six months of age. This would give them a good chance of entering first grade with sufficient communication skills to be able to benefit from school. Infants with risk indicators for progressive or delayed-onset hearing loss should receive audiological monitoring every six months until age three to make sure the audiologist and team of service providers are making necessary adjustments to help the child.

Hearing screening is a quick and virtually painless process. The two most commonly used methods are Automated Auditory Brainstem Response (AABR; see Figure 2.1) and Automated Otoacoustic Emissions (AOAE; see Figure 2.2). AABR (Erenberg, 1999) is easy to use, fast, cost-effective, and accurate. A nurse tapes a few electrodes to the baby's head, places a soft tip in the baby's ear, and then a machine makes clicking sounds. The electrode measures the baby's brain's response to the sounds. AOAE (Barker, Lesperance, & Kileny, 2000) tests the baby's inner ear, specifically the cochlea. Again, a soft tip is placed in the baby's ear, the equipment makes sounds, and the tip measures activity in the ear. Most states recommend procedures for hospitals to follow to make sure that any child who receives a positive rating for potential hearing loss is re-screened and then sent to the various service providers for appropriate help.

Although as a nation we are getting better at identifying children with hearing loss right out of the hospital, many children still are not identified until about age two, which used to be the traditional age of identification (Harrison, Roush, & Wallace, 2003). Many reasons account for this. First, newborn hearing screening may result in false negatives; that is, the test may show the child has normal hearing when he does not. Next, a progressive loss may be present and not show up until the baby is older. Further, mild losses may be more difficult to detect.

Unfortunately, there are also reasons why no follow-up to initial screening occurs. First, the newborn nursery staff may downplay the significance of poor results on a screening test. Second, parents may move from one town to another and drop out of the public tracking system's safety net. Third, parents may fear the findings of a follow-up test and may choose not to consider the loss until the child is older and it becomes more evident. In addition, some areas of the country do not offer these types of services or the parents may be newcomers to the United States who missed out on screening because the child was born in a hospital without newborn screening service. In some cases the child may have been born at home. When these children are identified and start the language learning process, they already have missed out on some key development milestones for communication acquisition.

Figure 2.1   Automated Auditory Brainstem Response

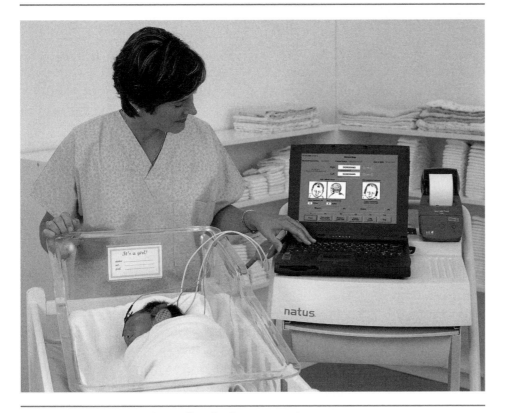

SOURCE: Image courtesy of Natus® Medical Incorporated.

Figure 2.2   Automated Otoacoustic Emissions

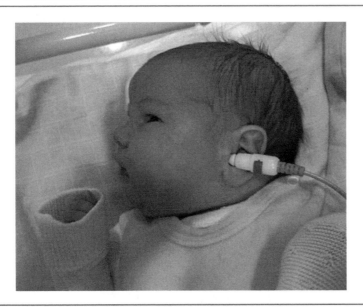

SOURCE: Image courtesy of Natus® Medical Incorporated.

NECESSARY SERVICES FOR INFANTS, TODDLERS, AND THEIR FAMILIES

When you work with a baby, you will need to call upon a multidisciplinary team (Gallagher, Easterbrooks, & Malone, 2006). Many organizations and agencies can provide services (see Resource A), so you will need to hone your collaboration skills. Get all the advice and assistance you can from all the sources you can. If one service says that you must work exclusively with them, question the wisdom of this. No one knows everything there is to know about every child. Consult with as many sources as you can. The Internet holds more information than you can possibly use. Use this as a tool to learn ways of helping your little one catch up to the skills of his hearing peers.

Find a good pediatric audiologist who can advise you on how to make the most out of the child's residual hearing (the child's remaining hearing). Very few babies are born profoundly deaf. Most have some sort of usable hearing. The audiologist is the best person to help determine how much hearing remains and how best to use technology, such as hearing aids and cochlear implants, to improve the child's hearing. ASHA publishes guidelines for pediatric assessments.

Help parents find a good program that has a history of working successfully with babies and toddlers who are deaf and hard of hearing. Most states have parent-infant programs (Arehart, Yoshinaga-Itano, Thomson, Gabbard, & Brown, 1998). Private schools and clinics in larger cities also can be valuable sources of information. These programs can provide appropriate assessment and intervention and can teach parents how to become the naturally communicating support system their child needs in order to develop language.

Obtain a comprehensive evaluation to help determine appropriate learning goals and target objectives. Get information about the child's hearing and use of hearing devices (see Chapter 6), his listening skills, speech skills, language skills, and other developmental skills. Other developmental skills include but are not limited to growth and health, cognition, and play skills. See Resource B for lists of age-appropriate assessment tools.

Federal law allows states to provide services to infants and toddlers with disabilities. In order to do so, a multidisciplinary team meets to develop an Individualized Family Service Plan (IFSP). The IFSP must contain information based on the assessments given to the child. The team identifies outcomes, or target objectives, during the IFSP meeting, as well as the criteria, procedures, and timeline for measuring progress. The team discusses methods and strategies that service providers will use, and identifies a service coordinator. The team considers ways that community agencies can help children and families (e.g., health, transportation, and child care). Finally, the team explores a plan to transition the child from early intervention services to preschool services in the local school system by age three. The IFSP team might consist of:

- An audiologist for consultation on acquiring and using listening devices such as hearing aids or cochlear implants

- Parent-infant support agencies for access to highly qualified teachers and speech-language pathologists

- Related service providers such as physical therapists, occupational therapists, and others who can assist with other aspects of a child's needs

- Social workers for assistance with financial and social aspects of accessing necessary support

As soon as the team identifies the necessary services and support systems, it is important to begin child and family intervention. The goal of universal newborn hearing screening is to have every infant with a hearing loss identified by three months of age and every family involved in child and family services by the time the child is six months of age (Joint Committee on Infant Hearing, 2000). Some babies receive services almost immediately after leaving the hospital. The earlier the team can establish the necessary services, the better (Yoshinaga-Itano, Sedey, Coulter, & Mehl, 1998). Table 2.1 lists services that the IFSP team should discuss.

Table 2.1   Services IFSP Teams Should Consider During a Team Meeting

Audiology Services
Otology and Geneticist Services
Awareness of Communication Options
Auditory-verbal, auditory-oral, various signed English options, American Sign Language
Communication Intervention
Specialized Therapies
Physical therapy, occupational therapy, auditory-verbal therapy, speech therapy
Family Counseling, Family Services, and Mental Health Services
Listening and Other Technology

SOURCES: Gallagher, Easterbrooks, and Malone (2006); Proctor, Niemeyer, and Compton (2005).

HOW LISTENING DEVELOPS IN INFANTS AND TODDLERS

Newborn babies respond to sounds around 40 to 50 dB (Eliot, 1999), primarily because their response systems have not developed yet. It's pretty amazing, then, that most parents have a natural tendency to speak more loudly and closer to their newborns. Newborns are sensitive to the prosody (sing-songiness) of their parents' or caregivers' voices. Older babies, in fact, will show a definite preference for the prosody of their native language over the prosody of a different language (Jusczyk, Friederici, Wessels, Svenkerud, & Jusczyk, 1993). This means that when you are working with a baby who has a hearing loss, you need to be in very close proximity, and you need to use *motherese*, the style of interaction that mothers use when talking to their babies. It includes a raised pitch, exaggerated prosody, repetition, shorter utterances, and a slower pace (see Table 2.2).

Once the baby reaches about six months of age, his threshold improves to about 20 to 25 dB (Eliot, 1999), not because he is hard of hearing, but because

Table 2.2 Characteristics of Motherese

Singsongy sounding

Mothers put all the suprasegmentals of spoken communication (duration, intensity, pitch) together in a singsongy voice for their babies. The emotional range of what a mother is saying is also reflected in this style (also called prosody).

Temporal resolution and lengthening sounds

Mothers slow down and lengthen their speech so that babies can grasp what they are saying. The developing brain takes a while to differentiate between sounds.

Memory constraints

Mothers speak in shorter phrases and sentences to account for the baby's developing memory skills.

In addition to motherese, early communication interactions should address reduced competition from noise. The world sounds like a wild and crazy place to a baby because she has not yet fine-tuned her listening skills by organizing sounds in her brain. Be sure to spend some of your involvement time every day in a quiet environment where the child can best access your voice without competition from the noisy world.

his brain has learned to hear fine-tuned differences. For example, babies are more sensitive to high-frequency sounds such as a tea kettle than to low-frequency sounds. This may be related to the fact that most mothers naturally tend to raise the pitch of their voices when talking to their babies, a feature of motherese. In essence, the brain is moving from being a nonlistener to a listener. Early intervention in the first six months should take advantage of this natural progression from confusion over what sounds mean to an understanding of them. By the time a child is in preschool, his hearing threshold is around 10 dB, and by the time a child is a teenager, his hearing has reached its potential, only to start the inevitable decline in the adult years (Eliot, 1999).

Temporal resolution, or the length of time it takes to hear a sound before we perceive it to be different from another sound, improves with time (Trainor, Samuel, Desjardins, & Sonnadara, 2001). For example, adults can distinguish sounds that differ by 1/100th of a second. A six-month-old baby needs to hear a sound for twice as long before he perceives it as different, and a six-year-old falls somewhere in the middle. This may be why mothers naturally speak more slowly to their babies, another feature of motherese.

As the newborn explores her world, myelination of the nerves (a protein coating that develops over time and acts much the same as the plastic coating around an electrical wire) is occurring, and the brain synapses are developing. Just as a baby learns to crawl before jumping, nerve pathways become faster and more efficient with age and practice. Finally, the auditory cortex of the brain becomes more "grown-up" as it receives auditory stimulation. Auditory stimulation is the fodder that feeds the system and allows it to develop. If the child does not receive auditory stimulation, his auditory system cannot grow and mature.

Finally, the baby's brain is learning to sort through all the noises of the world, which mask speech. Babies become much better at tuning out noises by age two, with development continuing until around age ten. This means that when you are working with a baby, you need to present sounds in an organized way, and you need to do this when there aren't many distractions around. This is another good reason to move closer to a baby when you are working on language development.

HOW INFANTS DEVELOP SPOKEN LANGUAGE

We cannot overemphasize the importance of identification and intervention in the first year of life; they are the keys to successful communication development in children with hearing loss (Calderon, 2000; Yohsinaga-Itano, Sedey, Coulter, & Mehl, 1998).The infant's auditory system is a dry sponge waiting for stimulation. If you wait until a child is older to begin stimulating the auditory system, then this child will need more intensive adult support to make appreciable gains because the auditory system has not learned to listen. Not only that, it has actually learned *not* to listen, and if we begin stimulation later, then the teacher, clinician, and parents will have to overcome the tendency *not* to listen, making it more difficult to make headway.

All children with hearing loss, including those using cochlear implants, require a combination of didactic (direct and therapeutic) and incidental teaching (McConkey-Robbins, 1998) in order to be most successful. A child's potential for incidental learning and generalization is greatest in the early years and slowly decreases with age. Very young children can benefit most from incidental language learning when it is facilitated by an adult (Desjardin, Eisenberg, & Hodapp, 2006) and when they have appropriate amplification; however, simply putting a listening device on a child addresses only one part of the process. Learning to listen and to talk requires extensive and intensive support. The longer you wait to start this support, the more didactic, time-consuming, and labor-intensive the process becomes.

"Language input sculpts the brain to create a perceptual system that highlights the contrasts used in the language, while de-emphasizing those that do not, and this happens *prior* to word learning. The change in phonetic perception thus assists word learning, rather than the reverse" (Kuhl, 2000, p. 103). This means that auditory stimulation creates the perceptual system that supports language learning prior to the development of words. Infants start out with brains wired to hear a great variety of speech sounds. As people talk to them, their auditory systems change and develop. The connections among neurons associated with the language around them become stronger. Any residual connections having to do with their potential to learn other languages automatically tend to drop into the background. For example, by around 12 months, Japanese children do not hear the *r/1* distinction, and if they want to learn English later in life, they must make a conscious effort to listen for the differences (Best, 1994; Flege, 1995). Thus, by the end of the first year, children with normal hearing have developed a filter that is distinctly tailored to help them develop language. If a baby who cannot hear has received appropriate amplification (assuming there are no extenuating reasons why he should not or could not be amplified, such as problems with the physical structure of the ear) and has had the opportunity to listen to sounds presented to him by his caregivers in a nurturing environment, then he, too, has potential to develop this filter system that allows *language uptake.* We specify uptake as opposed to input because we cannot put communication into a child's head. He must choose to attend to and take up the stimulus.

Babies are natural magnets for language, as you've probably noticed. Our job in the first year with babies who are deaf and hard of hearing is to offer sounds in a meaningful way that will allow communication to bypass the filter of poor hearing. This makes the baby more efficient as a language learner and sets the stage for language learning.

Figure 2.3   Baby and Daddy Talk About Shoes

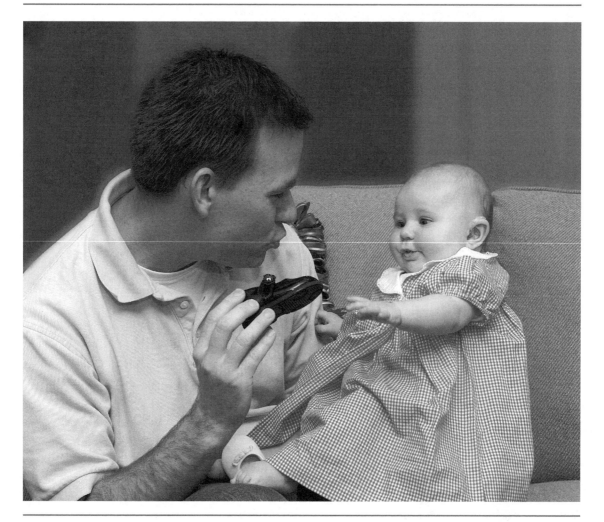

SOURCE: Photographed by John Zimmermann.

HOW TODDLERS DEVELOP SPOKEN LANGUAGE

By the time a child with normal hearing is around 18 months old, he has developed a vocabulary in the range of 50 to 100 words (www.fwspeech.com/milestones.php). The child understands very clearly that words can describe things, and he has an innate understanding that he can control and improve things in his life at a very practical level if he uses those words. He also develops the skill of novel mapping (Lederberg, Prezbindowsi, & Spencer, 2000). For example, if you place three objects in front of a child and he knows the word for two of them, and then you ask for the object that he doesn't know, he will give you that object because he understands that this new word must belong to the object for which he has no label. He is mapping a novel word onto something for which he does not have a word. It only takes this little guy one or two exposures to the word and, voila!—it's his.

Once most children begin novel mapping, they do it very fast (fast mapping), resulting in a vocabulary explosion. Some children aren't able to map as fast (slow mapping). As a result, their vocabulary development occurs at a more measured pace. Children with cognitive delays and children who have just been identified as having a hearing loss at 18 and 24 months of age are going to be slower mappers, and this will delay the process of language acquisition.

The most important tool we have for providing children with the material they need to learn language is *conversation*. The sheer number of words that a child is exposed to influences how well he will learn to communicate (Hart & Risely, 1995). When children have a hearing loss, they are deprived of the amount of listening hours in a manner similar to children from poorly communicating homes.

> In an average 14-hour waking day, a child spoken to 50 times per hour will hear 700 utterances, a child spoken to 800 times per hour will hear more than 11,000. Given the stability in family styles that we observed, it is staggering to think that 365 similar days in a year would produce in terms of cumulative experience with language and exposure to 250 thousand versus 4 million utterances. (Hart & Risely, 1995, pp. 70–71)

If the total number of utterances that a child hears results in a language user or nonuser, then we must be vigilant about bathing children in language at all times.

Another tool the child begins to use around this time is *pointing*. This helps him to clarify his words. For example, he might point to his bare feet and say "shoe," meaning that he doesn't have on his shoes. His parents or caregivers will say something like, "Shoes on? You want your shoes on?" Or, he might point to a doll whose shoe has fallen off, eliciting a response from his parents or caregivers such as, "Shoe off. Muffin's shoe fell off." Very shortly after the child starts to use this extremely important pointing bridge into early word-combining, we hear him saying, "Shoe on" or "Shoe off."

The pointing gesture, which happens with all children, is the hallmark of the *preinflected stage.* In the preinflected stage, children use two and three words with no inflections such as tense or number as in "My shoe on." Simultaneously, parents and caregivers are using lots of intonation. Their voices rise with question inflection when saying "shoe on?" but drop matter-of-factly when saying "shoe off." This does not go unnoticed by the child with typical hearing, who includes intonation with words to represent the basic declarative, interrogative, and exclamatory sentence types of communication— "Shoe?" "Shoe" and, "Shoe!"—all mean different things when coming out of the mouths of babes.

All babies use a pointing gesture as a means for bridging into better communication (Dobrich & Scarborough, 1984). However, some therapies expressly forbid a child to use his hands in any form of communication. This is not consistent with the language acquisition of children with normal hearing. All babies point before they use words, and they point as a bridge from single words to word combinations. Eliminating the source of information that links the child's thought or intention to the response he or she elicits from the parent, caregiver, teacher, or clinician violates a basic tenet of early intervention: to talk about the child's interests.

Recall that all of the above language learning can happen because the child with typical hearing is such a language magnet. When a child has just been identified with a hearing loss at age 18 months to two-and-one-half years, his brain has not yet developed this important foundation for language learning. Parents and caregivers must step back from "normal" language and work to assist the child in establishing this foundation.

Because the rest of the child's body has moved along in its development, we no longer have the nonambulatory little cutie pie bouncing in his pumpkin seat and listening, listening, listening to the world. Instead, we have an active

Figure 2.4   Toddler Points to Communicate

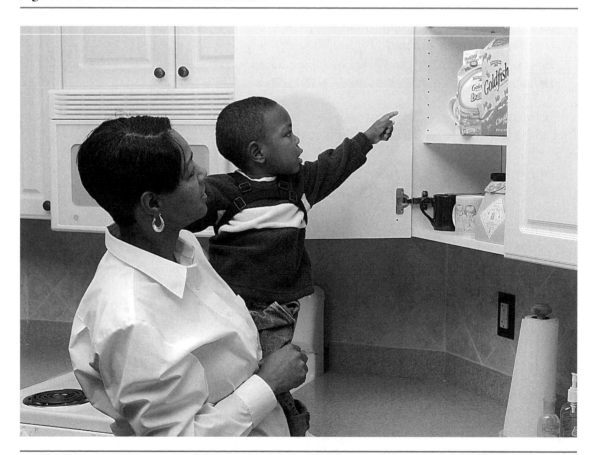

SOURCE: Photographed by John Zimmermann.

crawler, cruiser, walker, mover, jumper, thrower, digger, sniffer, biter, and grabber. The last thing this little one is going to sit still for is someone in his face with a singsongy voice. In order to get this child's attention, we will have to become much more engaging to compete with the world of doing that is now within his grasp. Making Sparky's food float in his water bowl is far more interesting than paying attention to someone saying, "Shoe, shoe. Here is your shoe." Sounds sculpt the perceptual system, so parents, caregivers, teachers, and clinicians need to learn ingenious ways of attracting and maintaining the toddler's attention. Because a toddler moves purposefully, we can more easily understand his intent. This gives us clues about the topics we should discuss. A toddler is aware that he can exhibit some control of the world. If we can

Table 2.3   Development of Early Communication Skills

Skill Area	Age
Speech or Phonological Skills	
Reflexive or precanonical vocalization	Birth to 6 weeks old
Cooing and laughter	6 to 16 weeks
Expansion stage	4 to 7 months
Growls, nasal murmur	
Single syllables with elongated vowels	7 to 10 months
Reduplicated or canonical babbling (e.g., gah, gah, gah)	
Engaging in sound play	
Variegated or nonreduplicated babbling (e.g, gah, boo, gah, bah)	11 to 18 months
Conversation babble and jargon	18 months to 2 years
True words	12 months
Language or Grammar Skills	
Pregrammatical one- and two-word utterances such as:	~ 18 months
Nouns, action words, modifiers, personal-social and functional words	
Primacy of nouns	
~ 50-100 words	
Noninflected three- and four-word utterances such as:	24 to 36 months
Simple conjunction, possession, entity, attributes, action, existence, recurrence (e.g., Daddy go work?)	
~ 200 + words	
Thinking Skills	
Discrimination, matching, imitation, making simple choices	~18 months
Sequencing two to three items or objects; organizing in space	24 to 36 months

SOURCES: Oller (1978); Owens (1996); Schumaker and Sheldon (1999).

teach a toddler that language can help him control his world, then we have a built-in motivator for the child to participate in our efforts. Table 2.3 identifies some of the major language and thinking skills that develop at very young ages.

INTERVENTIONS FOR BABIES

In the next section we list interventions that are appropriate to use when working with babies. Table 2.4 lists general suggestions that you should consider. We also relate additional suggestions to the *Model of Auditory, Speech, and Language Development* in Chapter 1.

Table 2.4   General Suggestions for Working With Infants

Fit the baby with a hearing aid as soon as possible, even if you are considering a cochlear implant when the child becomes eligible.

Much of what happens in the first year depends upon sensory stimulation. The amount of preverbal communication that a child uses (pointing, showing, responding, chattering, reaching, screaming, grunting, moving arms, etc.) and the frequency of communication are predictors of later communication success (Caselli, 1990). It doesn't matter whether the communication is gestural or vocal babble. Babies want responsive caregivers. Caregiver stimulation and the baby's own vocalizations help lay down neural tracks. Skipping this will only require greater compensatory effort later on.

Make your environment a stimulating one, including not only auditory stimulation but visual and tactile stimulation as well.

Sometimes we are so focused on developing the listening function that we forget that this is a whole child who is not only a listener but a watcher, a taster, a smeller, a thrower, and an all-round whole package.

Use natural visual gestures associated with communication.

All babies in all countries, both hearing and deaf, use natural gestures such as pointing as cues to parents and caregivers about what they want to know. Take advantage of these cues as they will help you talk about the child's interests.

Know when to include lipreading cues.

Hearing children depend on lipreading cues to help differentiate among sounds as they learn to listen. When working specifically on a new listening skill, cover your mouth, but in normal conversation, lipreading cues may be beneficial.

Increase your proximity to the baby.

Bring everything to the baby. Get up in his face and his line of vision. Put toys in his hands. Clap his hands together. Talk and sing directly to him. Hold him on your lap and talk to him. Bring the world of sensation to him.

Use motherese. Fathers can do this too.

Motherese (Fair, 1998) is that style of communication that hearing mothers use with babies who can hear and deaf mothers use with babies who are also deaf (see Table 2.2).

Recognize that parents have unique needs.

Parents may feel distanced from their baby, especially when the baby is nonresponsive. They may feel unsure about bonding. Parents can only go "on faith" for so long before they become frustrated. They need support and reassurance during no-response periods. They also need information. Children of parents who actively seek information tend to learn to communicate faster than those whose parents are reticent. Learn to recognize parent-child temperament mismatches and help them understand issues of child temperament.

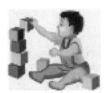

APPLYING THE *MODEL* WITH BABIES

Parameter 1: Brain Tasks

The primary brain task associated with little babies is detection. Focus all your efforts on bringing sounds to the child in an organized and meaningful way so that his brain will learn to detect them.

Parameter 2: Listening, Speaking, and Language Skills

Table 2.3 above summarizes the communication and thinking skills that babies and toddlers are developing. Your task is to encourage the baby to listen to you carefully so that she can discern the suprasegmentals, vowels, and consonants of spoken language. Ways that you can use to accomplish this include but are not limited to:

- Ellen Rhoades's *Sound-Object Associations* list (see newly revised version in Resource C). The sounds for the Sound-Object Associations list were chosen because they appear to be most helpful in exposing baby to various suprasegmentals, vowels, and consonants. For example, a toy cow or cow puppet can be used to expose baby to the "mooo" sound, which is a nasal consonant with a low-frequency sound. A toy cat or cat puppet can be used to expose baby to the "meow" sound, which combines a consonant and vowel, where the vowel is an easy-to-hear diphthong.

- Call the baby's attention to sounds at all times. Learn to use the "finger to ear" cue. Use this cue when you hear a sound and want to call it to baby's attention. You can gasp and have an excited look followed by pointing to your ear and then saying, "Airplane. Listen. I hear an airplane. Did you hear that? Aaaaaaaaa. There's an airplane." Use this cue any time there is a new sound introduced into your environment. Call your baby's attention to all the sounds you hear.

- Talk about everyday routines. There are dozens of things that you do on a daily basis and repeatedly throughout the day. Set up conversational routines and engage in your routine every time you do the activity. For example, when noticing that baby is wet say, "Uh-oh. You're wet. Time to change your diaper." After you put baby on the changing table say, "Diaper, let's change your diaper." When pulling off the sticky tabs say, "Pull. Oops. It's off! Pull again. Oops. It's off!" When removing the diaper say, "Off. Let's take your diaper off." Continue with this kind of monologue each time you change a diaper.

- Build up an anticipatory set. This will help your baby learn that sounds are forthcoming. When you know that a familiar sound is about to enter your environment, such as Grandpa walking through the door after work, say with excitement in your voice and on your face, "Listen. Grandpa is home. Where's Grandpa? I hear the door? Is that Grandpa? Yes, it's Grandpa!" Identify multiple times throughout the day or week when you can predict that there will be a sound, and then establish a routine of what to say. Some examples of these times include but are not limited to: the dog barking to come in, the delivery man ringing the doorbell, the buzzer on the washing machine about to buzz, and the engine of the car starting up.

Figure 2.5 Grandpa Walks Through Door and Greets Baby

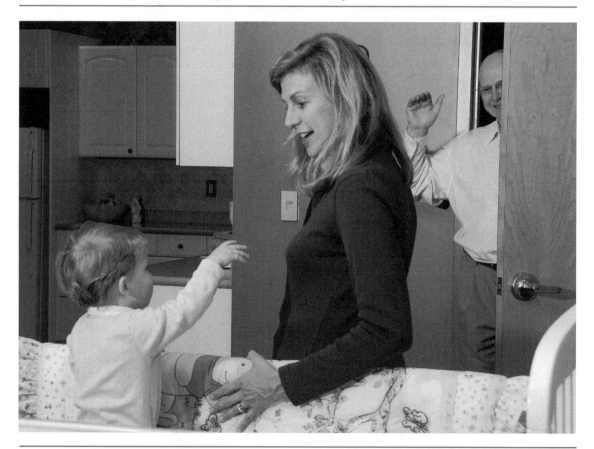

SOURCE: Photographed by John Zimmermann.

- Focus on age-appropriate vocabulary. The *MacArthur-Bates Communicative Development Inventory: Words and Gestures* (CDI; www.sci.sdsu.edu/cdi) lists the words used by infants from 8 to 16 months and provides a target vocabulary for parents, clinicians, teachers, and interventionists. Categories of identified vocabulary include: sound effects and animal sounds, animals (real or toy), other toys, food and drink, clothing, body parts, small household items, furniture and rooms, outside things and places to go, people, games and routines, action words, descriptive words, words about time, pronouns, question words, and quantifiers. The CDI Web site also provides normative tables for you to see which words are developing first in most babies and toddlers. It's best to begin to systematically expose babies to the words and sounds on the list.

- Use consonant-vowel combination mini-songs. Box 2.1 provides some sample mini-songs. A mini-song is a simple phrase repeated in a highly inflected, singsongy voice. While you are working through the Sound-Objects Associations list, you can also start using mini-songs to put sounds together in an organized sequence of vowel combinations. Vowels range from low to high contrast. Start with the vowels that have the greatest contrast in auditory, visual, and tactile feedback, and then move to finer distinctions.

Figure 2.6   Mother and Baby Play Horsey

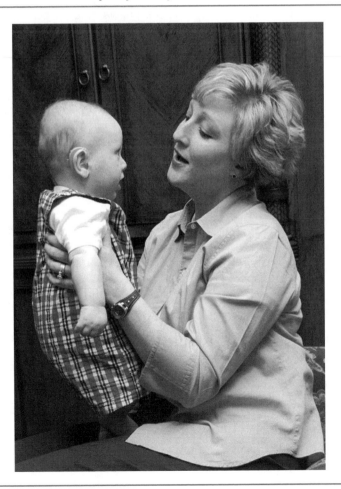

SOURCE: Photographed by John Zimmermann.

Box 2.1   Mini-Songs for Babies

Highest Contrast Examples

Go to bed

- Use this at bedtime or whenever your child goes down for her nap.
- Sing this: "Go to bed. Go to bed," as you and the child pretend to put her baby doll to sleep.
- Look through "The Three Bears," "The Seven Dwarfs," or any story when putting children to bed. Point out these pictures (and sing the phrase).

Take it

- When the toddler reaches for something, hand it to him and sing "take it!"
- When you are playing with toys, hand one to him and sing "take it!"

My cup

- Choose a special mug or cup that you will associate with this phrase all the time. When you are drinking coffee or tea, point out, "My cup, my cup. This is my cup."
- When you give baby a bottle say, "Here's your bottle. Here's my cup. My cup. Here's my cup."
- When washing dishes say, "My cup. See. I'm washing my cup."

- After the child has mastered single words and has listened to mini-songs, transfer listening skills to production of two-word semantic-syntactic pairs by facilitation techniques. Table 2.5 identifies early semantic-syntactic word pairs. Table 2.6 lists commonly used facilitation techniques.

Table 2.5   Early Semantic-Syntactic Word Pairs

Relation	*Example*
Agent + Action	Daddy bye-bye (Daddy is leaving.)
Negative + Entity	No bye-bye (I don't want Daddy to leave.)
Action + Location	Drive car (He is driving in the car.)
Entity + Location	Daddy office (Daddy is at the office.)
Possessive + Entity	Daddy car (Daddy's car)
Action + Recipient	Open me (Open the door for me.)
Introducer + Entity	That Daddy (There he is!)
Attribute + Entity	Happy Daddy! (He's so glad to see me!)
Action + Object	Kiss Daddy (Come here so I can give you a smooch!)

Table 2.6   Commonly Used Language Facilitation Techniques

Technique	Description
Expansion	Repeating utterance, retaining child's grammar and vocabulary, but enhancing accuracy
Expatiation	Repeating utterance and adding new information
Open-Ended Questions	Using simple wh- and yes/no questions surrounding actions and books
Parallel Talk	Talking about what the child is doing while he is doing it
Syntactic Recasting	Rephrasing a child's statement into a question
Semantic Recasting	Expanding a child's statement to invoke prior knowledge and evoke new connections

SOURCES: Desjardin, Eisenberg, and Hodapp (2006); Easterbrooks and Baker (2002).

Parameter 3: External Factors

When working with very young babies, external factors are easier to manage because you are bringing all objects and sounds to his attention. The stimulus array will for the most part be one item, one phrase, or one activity that you are asking him to pay attention to. Keep your linguistic complexity to short and simple words and phrases that you repeat again and again. Make the contextual environment very clear. Baby needs to hear, see, touch, feel, and taste everything that you are talking about while you are talking about it.

Parameter 4: Child Actions

What behaviors can we expect of a baby in response to the sounds that we provide? There are actually quite a few things that babies do to let us know that they are noticing things. They look, smile, flail their hands and arms, become quiet, gurgle and coo, quit sucking on a bottle, scrunch up their little faces, furrow their brows, and wiggle. Watch for these signs when your baby hears a sound.

INTERVENTIONS FOR TODDLERS

In this next section we list general suggestions to consider when working with a toddler (ten months to just under three years). Table 2.7 lists these suggestions. We also relate additional suggestions to the *Model* in Chapter 1. If the toddler has just been identified with a hearing loss, you will need to go back to the suggestions for babies and work through these processes and activities.

Table 2.7   General Suggestions for Working With Toddlers

Consider all the suggestions earlier in the chapter for working with infants.
Consider binaural amplification.

Use hearing aids or cochlear implants in both ears because older babies and toddlers are learning the important skill of localizing (i.e., finding the source) of sounds. This requires the use of two ears.

Continue to use natural visual pointing gestures to bridge to higher levels of grammar.

Use the words "look" and "see" often with a toddler to help him connect to the concepts that you are labeling.

Include lipreading cues where appropriate.

Place a toy in the child's line of sight; then draw her vision to your face to capitalize on lipreading cues.

Monitor proximity to the toddler's ear.

Toddlers are active, and your job will be to keep up with them. Squat down so that you are level with the hearing aids or cochlear implants, and then talk about your objective. Use fun objects and materials that capture their attention. Move it from the child's line of sight to your face. Then point to the child's ears and encourage her to listen to you. Talk and sing to her. Hold her in your lap and talk to her. Play lap games like "Ride the horsey. Ride to town." Follow her around and talk about everything she is interested in.

Continue to use motherese.
Expect plateaus.

This is normal and natural. Toddler development occurs at differing rates. One week they may be making a huge spurt in communication, and the next they may be learning to walk or jump. Be patient and keep up the conversation.

Help parents manage competing demands on their time.

Help parents brainstorm solutions to time challenges. If competing demands are not the problem, then discuss whether something about the early intervention process makes them uncomfortable. Be open and honest about this and ask how you can help.

Use nursery rhymes, fingerplays, and other verbal games that incorporate auditory closure.

This allows you to establish an anticipatory set, or expectation, for information the child is to fill in. For example, stress "snow" at the end of the first line of "Mary Had a Little Lamb." At the end of the second line, draw out "the lamb was su-u-re to _____" and encourage the toddler to complete (or close) the sentence.

Model linguistic interactions.

Have two adults model new skills. For example, if the child has trouble remembering to say "thank you," give another adult an object and have the second adult say "thank you" in an animated manner, using excited facial expression and a singsongy voice.

Use melodic intonation.

This is an exaggerated form of motherese by which you identify specific song patterns for common phrases and new language objectives. For example sing, "Good MOR-ning" several times when you first see the child in the morning or, "Cleeeean up! Cleeeean up!" when it is time to pick up toys.

Monitor "wait time."

Because toddlers must think about what they hear, they need extra time. We have a tendency to want to answers our own questions. When you have the urge to answer or prompt the child, count to 10, and then proceed. Some children need longer thinking time than this, so be ready to expand your comfort zone.

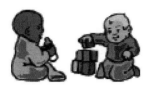

APPLYING THE *MODEL* WITH TODDLERS

Parameter 1: Brain Tasks

The primary brain task associated with recently diagnosed toddlers is detection. The brain tasks associated with toddlers who have been learning to listen for several months are detection, discrimination, and early work on identification of sounds. Focus all your efforts on bringing sounds to the child in an organized and meaningful way so that his brain will learn to detect, discriminate, and identify.

Parameter 2: Listening, Speaking, and Language Skills

Toddlers who are new to the listening, speaking, and language process will begin with all of the skills, strategies, and suggestions described above in the section on babies. You will also need to focus carefully on pattern practice associated with the suprasegmentals of speech. The toddler who has been listening for a while will be ready to start working on phrases and simple connected discourse. In addition to the strategies described under the babies section, you will work on the following:

- Pattern practice. Children need to listen to and discriminate different sound patterns based on the suprasegmentals of speech. Patterns of duration include short versus long (e.g., hop versus moooo), loud versus soft (e.g., STOP! versus shhhhhh), and low versus high (e.g., mooo versus peep-peep). Patterns of duration can vary based on single syllables, words with more than one syllable, or phrases with multiple syllables (e.g., "Don't cry" versus "Hug the puppy"). Begin by having the child listen to highly disparate patterns (e.g., "No" versus "Pour the milk"). As the child's listening ability improves, make the patterns you are asking him to compare more and more similar. Various curriculum guides and materials have suggestions for pattern practices. See Resource D for commercially available materials.

- Continue working on the words found in the MacArthur-Bates CDI's infant version and start to work on the words and sentences identified in the MacArthur-Bates CDI: Words and Sentences version, which is designed for toddlers, ages 16 to 30 months. In addition to the categories of vocabulary listed in the Babies section, this form expands to articles, helping verbs, and connecting words. Toddlers need a large vocabulary that contains a variety of nouns, verbs, adjectives, adverbs, and prepositions—the building blocks of grammar. Grammar development will occur more naturally if the child has a large lexicon of words to put together.

- Consonant vowel combination mini-songs. By the time the child is nearing her third year, you should be working on low contrast examples. Box 2.2 presents sample high and low contrast mini-songs for toddlers.

- Work on expanding word pairs (see Table 2.5) into larger phrases to develop the child's grammar. Also work on negation, contraction, question forms, and pronouns.

- Be sure when working on vocabulary that you present age-appropriate multiple meanings of words. For example, the toddler should know the difference between the action verb *run* and the adjective use *runny nose.*

Parameter 3: External Factors

External factors become very important when working with toddlers because a toddler is easily stimulated by all the exciting and new things in his environment. It's important to work hard to make sure that the environment supports the toddler's ability to pay attention. The stimulus array will start with one item, one phrase, or one activity that you ask him to pay attention to. Increase the number in the stimulus array by age. A two-year-old who is an experienced listener should be able to sort between two stimuli; an almost three-year-old can start listening to and discriminating among three sounds. Be sure to work with the child in quiet locations until he develops a good listening foundation. Toddlers benefit greatly from context and in fact are still perceptually bound to it. Be careful not to have too many competing stimuli in the environment or this naturally curious little creature will be diverting your plans before you know it.

Parameter 4: Child Actions

Toddlers can stop, go, push, pull, take, make, throw, catch, copy, place, and engage in a variety of large motor (movement) and small motor activities to let us know when they hear or discriminate between sounds. The more you can focus your activities on physical behaviors that are most natural for toddlers, the better able you will be to garner and maintain their attention as well as measure and document their progress.

IF A CHILD IS NOT MAKING MEASURABLE PROGRESS

- Recheck amplification. You may need a new device, or it may need remapping or reprogramming. Check battery, earmolds, and all parts.

- Keep track of the amount of time you are realistically devoting to verbal interactions with the toddler and then call on others to help you increase the amount of language available to the child.

- Make sure you are not moving too fast and trying to accomplish too much at once. Carefully structure the sounds, words, and language you are presenting.

Box 2.2   Mini-Songs for Toddlers

Highest Contrast Examples

Go to bed

- Use this target as you put dollies to bed.
- Play a color matching game. Color and cut out ten little beds. Color and cut out ten little babies wrapped in blankets. Match the colored blankets to the same color bed. When your child makes a match say, "Go to bed little baby. Go to bed."

Open the letter

- Let your child open your mail every day. Use the phrase repeatedly.
- Make mailboxes out of shoeboxes. Color or decorate them. Write "Mommy"on one box and the child's name on another. Send letters back and forth to each other.

Medium Contrast Examples

Thank you

- Say "thank you" anytime the child gives you something. Enlist the aid of your family. Encourage them to say "thank you" to the child when he passes a requested dish.
- Accept toys from the child. Have the child give you a toy and place it in your lap. Say, "thank you" each time. Repeat until the child gets the idea. Switch roles. Hand him a toy and encourage him to say "thank you."

Cat food

- Go to the grocery store and point out cans of cat food.
- Get a little stuffed kitty cat or kitty cat puppet. Pretend the puppet is eating cat food and say, "Cat food. Eat the cat food."

Low or No Contrast Examples

Pat, pat

- At nap time pat your baby on the back. Say "Pat, pat, pat," in a sing-songy voice.
- After bath, dab a powder puff into some loose powder and pat it on your arms, legs, and tummy. Say, "Pat, pat, pat. Pat your tummy. Pat your knees. Pat, pat."

Dance, dance

- Dance around the room saying, "Dance, dance, dancey dance."
- Make your dolls dance. As you move their little legs say, "Dance, dancey, dance."
- Make a puppet out of your hand. Make the letter "V" with your fingers and use them as legs. Draw a face on the back of your hand, and then let your hand puppet dance while you sing "Dancey dance."

- Work with a speech-language pathologist or teacher of the deaf who can help you interpret the child's audiogram so that you are choosing sounds that are available to the child and vocabulary and grammar that are appropriate for his developmental level.

- Document that you are choosing appropriate objectives (audible, not too many listening tasks at once).

Note if the child is naturally developing more dependence on visual interactions with others. This may indicate that you have not chosen the appropriate auditory stimuli and that you should be incorporating more visual cues such as lipreading and gestures. In other children it may mean that they would benefit from signed communication. If the latter is the case, work with an early interventionist who can help you support American Sign Language.

Assuming that all is going well with health, amplification, and consistent intervention, if the child has not made measurable differences in a three-month time span, add in visual language support such as lipreading, cues, or sign language. Sometimes a child will need to learn a skill through his visual system, and then he can master it in his auditory system. Not all children are able to become users of spoken communication. This is not something to leave up to chance or to take a "wait and see" attitude about. The charge to teachers, clinicians, and parents is to document his rate of auditory progress and to come to an agreement early on regarding the indicators that they will use to make the decision to switch to sign language.

THE NEED FOR FLEXIBLE MODELS

Much emphasis is placed today on intervention in naturalistic environments (Dunst & Bruder, 2002). A naturalistic environment is any environment where a baby or toddler finds himself for large periods of the day. This may be at home with a parent or in-home caregiver, at the home of a caregiver, or at a day care center. Preparing the parents to be interventionists is all well and good, but what happens when the child spends most of his hours in a day care center? In this case it is important for individuals responsible for the child to receive the training alongside the parents.

We believe that limiting intervention to the home environment is not appropriate in all cases. Sometimes parents or caregivers are unable to completely implement the suggestions of an advisor. Some parents don't have the mind-set to be their child's teacher. Some parents may believe that they should be allowed to be a parent rather than an interventionist and may need additional support. Some mothers have several children and are unable to find the time in a day to provide the appropriate amount of intervention. Others may not have the temperament to work with their babies. Also, socio-cultural differences may arise when families have a different home language and home culture from the school or clinic.

The interventionist must understand the cultural implications of an outsider working within the home of someone whose culture sets parameters on who may do what in their homes. In addition, parents' objectives for their child cannot be overlooked. If the objective is for the child to learn spoken English, then a naturalistic environment in which English is not spoken will not promote that objective. Because early intervention programs in many states fall under the auspices of public health, a deaf education professional may not be involved in the case. If there are no alternatives to naturalistic environments, then what becomes of this baby? In these situations it becomes necessary to seek advice from a center or school where there is an appropriate educator (Arehart & Yoshinaga-Itano, 1999).

SUMMARY

This chapter presented information on universal newborn hearing screening, services needed by infants and toddlers with hearing loss and their families, development at this stage, and developmentally appropriate interventions. To summarize, we suggested that teachers:

- Call in the troops! Get all the outside help you can find.

- Find a good, qualified pediatric audiologist.

- Find a good program of early intervention support.

- Obtain a comprehensive listening, language, speech, and other developmental evaluation so that you will know what the child can do and needs to learn.

- Develop an Individualized Family Service Plan, including a transition plan.

- Begin child intervention immediately.

- Begin family intervention immediately.

Interventions for Preschoolers 3

In this chapter we describe interventions for preschoolers from age three to kindergarten entry. The main objectives for this chapter are to describe how to create a strong auditory learning environment and how to plan and implement auditory experiences in the preschool setting that will support a child's continued spoken language development.

When a child reaches preschool age, he is ready to socialize. He is also ready to control his environment through language. A child with a hearing loss who has been properly served in an early intervention program has a good head start on these skills. The preschool teacher will build on that foundation and will continue to encourage communication development during the preschool years. A child who is entering preschool with no spoken language skills needs a supportive environment to establish the skills discussed in Chapter 2 and to build a solid language foundation.

COLLABORATING WITH SERVICE PROVIDERS

When working with children who have a hearing loss, your first job is to call in the experts. No two deaf or hard of hearing children are alike. Necessary services may range from typical prekindergarten placement to special classes for deaf children only, along with a variety of related services. The early interventionist who worked with the child and her family before the child turned three can be of considerable help here. This person may work with a state agency, or may come from a private school or clinical program. Make an appointment right away to pick this person's brain. As you collaborate, be sure to get answers to all the questions shown in Table 3.1. In the next section, we will explain why this type of information is important in providing appropriate services.

Table 3.1   Questions Every Teacher Should Ask About a Child With Hearing Loss

Questions to Ask About the Hearing Loss

1. What kind of hearing loss does the child have, and how might it affect speech perception?
2. Is the child's loss unilateral or bilateral?
3. Is the child's loss fluctuating and/or progressive?
4. What is the cause of the child's hearing loss?
5. At what age did the child acquire the hearing loss?

Questions to Ask About Previous Intervention

1. At what age did the child start wearing hearing aids and receiving intervention?
2. What objectives were mastered relative to the *Model of Auditory, Speech, and Language Development* (Figure 1.1) during the years prior to preschool?
3. What kind of early intervention did the child and his family receive and how much?

Question to Ask About Listening Technology

1. What type of listening technology does this child use?

Questions to Ask About the Child With No Prior Services

1. How do I incorporate early-developing goals with the advanced cognitive level of the child?
2. How do I meet the needs of the parents to further their ability to help their child progress?

Questions to Ask About Learning Challenges

1. How do the additional learning challenges (e.g., vision) impact the child's perception and factor into my planning for stimulation?

WHAT YOU NEED TO KNOW ABOUT A CHILD'S HEARING LOSS

Type of Hearing Loss

You will want to know if the child's hearing loss is conductive, sensorineural, or mixed in order to make sure the parents understand whether they need to take any audiological or medical actions. Some malformations of the ear are treatable with surgery; some are not. Sometimes people will erroneously wait until surgery is completed before worrying about hearing aids. This is wrong. The child needs to be fitted with appropriate hearing aids until surgery can be performed. If not, you will miss valuable time during which the child could be using his hearing to promote spoken language development.

If otitis media (i.e., an active ear infection or fluid in the ears) is causing the hearing loss, you will need to take steps to help the family get the child proper medical care. A child with otitis media usually feels poorly because he has a cold or allergies, or his ear hurts. On top of that, he may have a hearing loss that prevents him from hearing as well as he could. Warning signs of otitis media include tugging on the ear, runny nose, general fussiness and saying, "Huh?" a lot. If you're listening carefully, you may notice a change in the child's speech patterns as he omits or distorts the pronunciation of sounds he no longer hears. Otitis media should be treated immediately. Malformation of the ear and middle ear problems are conditions that can lead to conductive hearing loss. These conditions are vastly improved when the child is fitted with a hearing aid that amplifies sound.

A child with a sensorineural hearing loss will not hear sound clearly no matter how loud the sound is. Depending on the degree of the hearing loss (explained in the next section), the child may function quite well with hearing aids, or he may require a cochlear implant to understand speech. A cochlear implant would not be indicated for children with no cochlea. Some children may have auditory dyssynchrony (also called auditory neuropathy), where the message does not seem to make its way up the auditory nerve. This condition has varying degrees of effect. Careful stimulation, observation, planning, and follow-up are necessary to determine the appropriate intervention for a child with auditory dyssynchrony.

Finally, children can have a mixed loss, which describes the case in which a child has both a conductive and sensorineural cause for the hearing loss. If the conductive component is caused by bouts of otitis media, teachers will need to adjust their teaching strategies to accommodate the child's needs during these occurrences of diminished perception.

Degree of Hearing Loss

You will want to know whether the child's loss is minimal, profound, or somewhere in between. The reason is because different degrees of loss cause the child to respond differently to sounds. Most professionals specify the "degree" or ranges of hearing loss as *minimal* (16–25 dB), *mild* (26–40 dB), *moderate* (41–55 dB), *moderate to severe* (56–70 dB), *severe* (71–90 dB), and *profound* (91+ dB). In general, the greater the hearing loss, the more significant impact it will have on the child's development of skills and competencies. For example, a child with a mild hearing loss will be able to understand most words in a sentence when listening in a quiet environment and will likely have speech that is clear and easy to understand. The child will have difficulty hearing some quiet sounds such as /s/ and /t/, and may not use morphological constructions such as plural –*s* or past tense –*ed* (see Chapter 6 for more information on morphology). He may mispronounce some words, have trouble hearing when there's background noise, and misunderstand the teacher.

A child with a profound hearing loss, on the other hand, will be able only to hear the first formant of vowels and some of the voiced consonants (see Chapter 6 for information on vowel formants). This child will not understand speech through listening alone, unless it is presented in very structured, quiet situations, using stimuli that are very distinct auditorily. This child may have a distinct vocal quality, different sounding from a child with normal hearing her same age. She may have a voice that is uniformly high or low pitched. She may mispronounce most speech sounds including vowel sounds. While mispronunciation of the vowels sounds is very rare in children with normal hearing, it is quite common in children with severe and profound hearing losses.

> ## Amy
>
> Amy is three years old. She is profoundly deaf and has just recently received a cochlear implant. She has no additional disabilities. She received early intervention and has a modicum of sign language that is phasing out in favor of auditory stimulation. Amy has a tendency to answer impulsively, repeating what the teacher has said without really listening. The teacher understands what she is saying as long as the context is high but misunderstands her in low context situations. Amy works individually with a speech-language pathologist for 45-minute sessions, three times each week, but therapy is not going well because Amy does not know the vocabulary underlying the speech lessons.
>
> Children like Amy need to develop a key vocabulary rapidly. Due to Amy's age, instruction should include the use of real objects rather than pictures. Amy also needs to learn how to make choices rather than answering impulsively. She may need to start at an easier listening task and build her ability to handle the current lessons. Most likely she needs to work on perceiving pattern differences such as "ahhhhhhh" for airplane and an intermittent (staccato) sound such as "ruff, ruff, ruff" for a dog rather than producing speech. This distinction relies on duration cues, not frequency cues. If Amy cannot discriminate between them after a week of practice, the teacher should contact the implant audiologist to get Amy's implant program reconfigured (remapped). The teacher needs to make sure that she provides lots of context cues so that she will understand Amy and Amy will understand her.

Laterality of the Loss

You will want to know if your student's loss is unilateral or bilateral in order to determine where to stand or sit relative to the child and whether he will need one hearing aid or two. A unilateral hearing loss is one where the child has normal hearing in one ear and a hearing loss in the other. A child with a unilateral hearing loss may benefit from having a hearing aid and/or assistive listening device fit on the ear with the hearing loss. Children with unilateral hearing losses have difficulty understanding where sound is coming from (localizing) and understanding speech in noisy environments. As a result, they can be accused of having behavior problems due to the effects of the hearing loss. An audiologist will need to closely follow children with unilateral hearing losses because some etiologies (causes) of unilateral losses result in eventual loss of hearing in both ears.

A child with a *bilateral hearing loss* often has a different level of hearing in each ear. The audiologist will have programmed the hearing aid or cochlear implant to fit the specific degree and shape of the hearing loss in each ear. It is crucial to know which device to use on which ear. Be sure you have correct and current information from the audiologist. It's a good idea to mark the devices or settings with a sticker or permanent ink to help you quickly know which one goes with which ear.

Stability of the Loss

You will want to know if your child's loss is progressive or fluctuating. A progressive loss is one in which the child's hearing worsens over time. A fluctuating hearing loss is one in which the hearing level changes up and down in an irregular manner. For example, the hearing loss can be in the moderately severe range one day and shift to the severe to profound range the next. If a child has a fluctuating loss, he will hear better on some days than others, and you will want to make sure your instruction accommodates the shift in hearing (e.g., providing visual cues, reducing the difficulty of external factors) and that you re-teach the information he missed on his "bad hearing" days. If a child has a progressive hearing loss, you will need to watch for signs of worsening hearing so you can encourage the parents to take the child to a doctor or audiologist.

A child with a progressive or fluctuating hearing loss requires close monitoring by an audiologist and detailed communication among the members of the educational team. Children with fluctuating or progressive hearing losses should be retested routinely to keep a close eye on the pattern and progress of changes in hearing acuity. People who work with the child need to keep close track of behavioral changes (such as acting out, or saying, "Huh?" a lot) and physical changes (such as loss of balance or dizziness). These changes can indicate a shift in the child's hearing level and would indicate a need for a trip to the audiologist or to the child's doctor.

Cause of the Loss

You will want to know the cause of the child's hearing loss because different etiologies have different implications for intervention. For example, if a child has lost his hearing due to an infection involving the brain, he may also have additional learning challenges that will need to be addressed. If a child's hearing loss is hereditary, it is less likely there will be concomitant disorders. The etiology of a hearing loss can provide information about how well the child hears and what management might be appropriate.

Age of Acquisition of the Loss

You will want to know at what age the child acquired the hearing loss because the older the child is when she loses her hearing, the more language she may have. A child who was born with a hearing loss doesn't have any experience with sound. Her brain hasn't had a chance to begin filtering for sounds and developing speech perception. If a child acquired a hearing loss or has a progressive loss that did not become profound until after she developed some language skills (postlingual), she will likely have some memory for speech that you will be able to enhance.

WHAT YOU NEED TO KNOW ABOUT PREVIOUS INTERVENTION

Age of Intervention and Age at Which Child Received Listening Technology

The number of months/years between when the child received his hearing aids or cochlear implants and the child's current age is called the child's "listening age." For example, if a child first received his hearing aids when he was 18 months old and he is currently age four-and-one-half years, his listening age would be three years. Knowing a child's listening age will allow you to plan instruction at auditory and language levels that are appropriate for his listening age while at the same time stimulating at a cognitive level appropriate for his chronological age.

It is also helpful to know the length of time the child did not have useable hearing (duration of deafness). This information will influence the child's rate of progress and could influence your decisions about appropriate expectations. A child who does not receive appropriate listening technology until the age of five or six and has no memory for sound (i.e., did not have a progressive or acquired hearing loss) will require much more therapeutic-type intervention than stimulation in the naturalistic environment associated with a classroom. This child will need stimulation following the *Model of Auditory, Speech, and Language Development* in Chapter 1 and going through the stages outlined in Chapter 2.

It is often helpful to keep track of a child's listening age during the first two or three years of intervention. When evaluating the child, compare her scores to the norms at her listening age in addition to her chronological age. Her scores should be in the average range when compared to her listening age. As the intervention progresses, she should make at least the same amount of progress that a child with normal hearing would make. She needs to make even greater strides in her skills to close the gap between her scores based on her listening age and her scores based on her chronological age. After the child has been in intervention for more than three years, the statistic of listening age is no longer meaningful; rather, we want to compare this child to her chronological age-mates.

Auditory, Speech, and Language Objectives Mastered During Preschool Years

You will want to know the child's present levels of performance in listening, speaking, and language. This will allow you to begin working immediately at appropriate instructional levels. During preschool years, early interventionists tend to allow the natural language of play-based experiences to guide their choice of vocabulary and concepts to teach. When a child has a hearing loss, we need to be purposeful and detailed in determining what skills to present. There is a difference between the skills you will incorporate into the naturalistic experiences of a preschool classroom and the skills you target for direct instruction. Often, it is simply a matter of structured and sufficient exposure for children with normal hearing to acquire new speech and language skills. However, we cannot be that unstructured with children with hearing losses. Adequate information about present levels of performance and strengths and weaknesses are necessary to help you plan your course of action. You will also want to know the level of structure that was necessary for his prior intervention to be effective.

Your intervention program will always require built-in family support. Some families will enter the preschool years with a lot of information about how to help their child continue to develop. Some families, on the other hand, may erroneously feel their part in the language development adventure is over when in fact it needs to continue full-steam ahead. The more support a family receives the more likely you can count on their involvement in the future. Parents who have not had the benefit of early intervention may still be dealing with some of the frustrations and confusion that arise surrounding the deaf or hard of hearing child. Your job will be to help parents as well as their children. Being aware of prior services received will help you determine where to begin.

Bryan

Bryan is almost four-and-a-half years old. He has a severe hearing loss and has worn hearing aids for two years. He has been receiving intervention services since he was two and a half. He attends a self-contained preschool class for children who are deaf or hard of hearing. He is in an auditory-oral classroom. There is no sign language used in the classroom. The teacher is a certified teacher of the deaf and hard of hearing. She is working with him on perceiving the differences between initial consonants. The teacher uses the words: *mat, cat, rat, hat,* and *bat.* Applying the *Model of Auditory, Speech, and Language Development* (Figure 1.1), the goal would look like this: Bryan will demonstrate identification (brain task) of single-syllable words differing by consonants (listening and speaking skill—consonants) when in the initial position of words (external factor—linguistic complexity) presented in a set of five objects (external factor—stimulus array) by pointing to pictures.

A four-and-a-half year old is typically old enough to recognize that pictures represent real objects; however, pictures should be realistic. The teacher needs to be sure Bryan knows these words before beginning this task. If he doesn't, the teacher must incorporate a vocabulary lesson into the session, or teach these words in another context before presenting them in this way. Regarding the word *hat,* the teacher is careful to use a picture of a hat and not a cap, such as a baseball cap. Calling a baseball cap a "hat" artificially restricts vocabulary growth. Knowledge of Bryan's vocabulary level helps the teacher choose the activities.

WHAT YOU NEED TO KNOW ABOUT LISTENING TECHNOLOGY

Type of Technology Used

You will need to know what type of listening technology your child uses so you can consult the best resources to properly use and maintain it. Your child could be using a hearing aid, a cochlear implant, an individual assistive listening device, and/or a sound field system at any one time. You must know the proper settings and programs for these devices. An audiologist will set each program to modify the sound signal in a different way. For example, the child might have a special program for listening in noisy situations and another one for listening in quiet. Audiologists often put multiple programs on cochlear implants and will ask you to try the different programs for a period of time and monitor the child's reactions to the sounds. This is especially true with children who have recently received the implant. The audiologist may load programs that gradually make the signal stronger or emphasize a particular aspect of sound. The audiologist will have a plan for when to use each program. The audiologist will benefit greatly from your feedback about how the child is responding to sounds.

Hearing aids, cochlear implants, and assistive listening devices have volume controls and other settings that you need to monitor. If you don't receive information from the audiologist about the proper settings on all of the devices the child is using, it is your responsibility to get that information. It is also your responsibility to make sure you have permission from the parents to contact the audiologist. Close communication with your child's audiologist is of paramount importance.

Carmen

Carmen is four. She has a moderate hearing loss in the low frequencies that slopes down to a profound hearing loss in the high frequencies. Every day she comes into the special needs class for children with varying exceptionalities and the teacher helps her take off her hearing aids and put on her individual FM system. During the middle part of this particular morning, the teacher is working with four other children, so she directs Carmen to color or look at books in the back of the classroom with some other children. Carmen leaves the table and pulls the blocks down off the shelf behind her. The teacher calls her name, but she does not look up. The teaching assistant walks over to Carmen and scolds her for not listening. Carmen has a temper tantrum and is put in time-out. After time-out, the teacher tries to talk to Carmen and notices that the FM system is not turned on. Carmen has not been able to hear anything since the moment the FM system was put on her, two hours earlier.

Fortunately for Carmen, the teacher recognized the problem with Carmen's assistive listening device. If she had not, Carmen could have spent her entire day with her FM system turned off. The teacher resolves to be more diligent in monitoring the device and asking for assistance in learning strategies to employ when Carmen does not respond. Carmen might have been labeled a behavior problem when all she really had was an equipment problem. Appropriately, this teacher called for help from members of the multidisciplinary support team.

WHAT YOU NEED TO KNOW ABOUT A CHILD WITH NO PRIOR SERVICES

When a child comes to preschool with no prior intervention, that child enters at a significant disadvantage. Start by rereading all the information on strategies at the infant and toddler level. You are just now starting the intervention clock for this child. What listening and language skills would you expect of a six-month-old? That is what you can expect from the preschooler six months from the day you first initiate intervention. The clock starts ticking when the child receives his first hearing aid and when the adults in his environment start interacting in a manner supportive of speech, listening, and language development. Rely on all of the other members of the multidisciplinary team to help you. Hard work is in store for all of you!

It is also essential to know whether the child has additional learning challenges or not. Visual, physical, cognitive, emotional, or medical conditions add to the needs of an already challenged child and may influence which strategies you choose.

PLANNING AND IMPLEMENTING INSTRUCTION AND INTERVENTIONS

The goal of auditory stimulation of young children with hearing loss is for listening to become integrated into the child's personality and to be as meaningful a source of information as vision and all other senses. Even though her hearing may be degraded compared to a person with normal hearing, she should rely on her hearing abilities as completely as she relies on her other senses.

There are two parts to auditory learning: auditory lessons and auditory experience. These two interventions have distinct characteristics and purposes. Auditory lessons are highly structured while auditory experiences are naturalistic.

Auditory Language Lessons

Auditory lessons focus on specific targets in structured situations. Auditory lessons develop new skills and expand existing ones. These tasks require high levels of concentration and effort from the child. You should use these times to stretch the child's abilities to the next level. Here is an example of an auditory lesson according to the *Model of Auditory, Speech, and Language Development* (see Figure 1.1). *Isaac will demonstrate identification (brain task) of single-syllable words with varying vowels and consonants (listening and speaking skill) when in the context of four critical elements (external factor of stimulus) by correctly choosing the animal named (child action).* The teacher would name one of the animals in the array such as "cow" or "horse." Isaac would repeat the word, pick up the animal, and interact with it in some way (such as making it walk across the table). To expand an existing listening and speaking skill, the teacher might put it in a more complex linguistic environment (such as embedding the skill in a phrase by saying, "Give me the horse" or "Put the horse on the floor," instead of just saying "horse"). Try to conduct the auditory lessons in a quiet room, free from distractions, and no more than a few children. Structured auditory lessons must be meaningful so that the child will learn that listening has a purpose.

Auditory Language Experiences

Auditory experiences happen naturally throughout the day although they may require deliberate effort from the teacher to set up. These situations require

Figure 3.1   Isaac Participates in a Structured Auditory Language Lesson

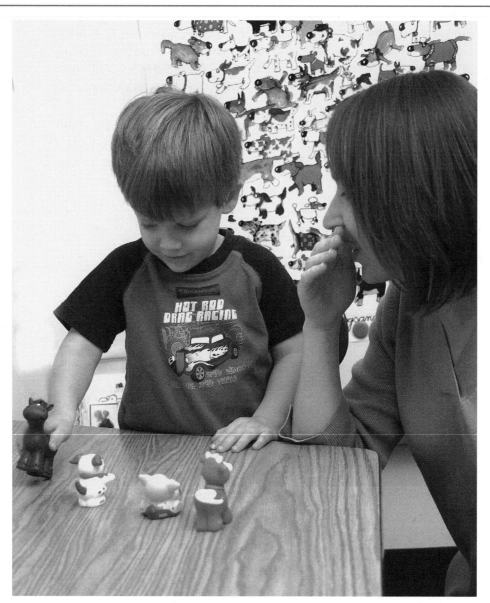

SOURCE: Photographed by John Zimmermann.

less focused effort on the part of the child and serve to foster dependence on hearing. Take advantage of all the opportunities that arise to communicate through audition as were described in Chapter 2 (i.e., knocking on door, sitting and looking at a book). For example, Ansley is just starting to respond to sounds, so when someone starts hammering on the other side of the wall, the therapist would stop the activity with a look of surprise and say, "Listen! I hear something! Let's go see what that is!!" Ansley and the therapist would find the person who is hammering, talk with that person about why, and then go back to the room. Upon returning to their room and hearing the sound again, the therapist would acknowledge the sound and help Ansley make the connection to the activity happening on the other side of the wall. One purpose of this natural auditory experience is to establish a spontaneous response to sound.

Figure 3.2   Isaac Participates in a Naturalistic Auditory Language Experience

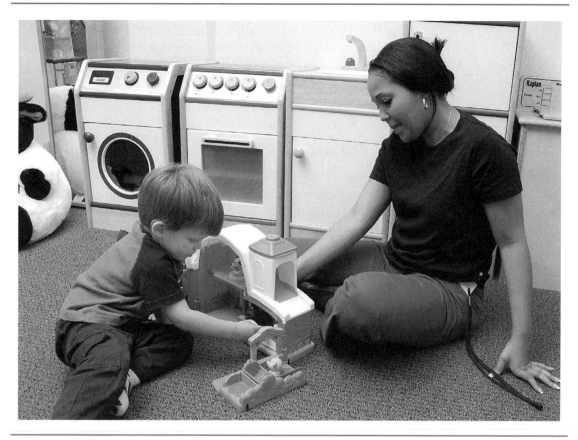

SOURCE: Photographed by John Zimmermann.

Mode of Presentation

Spoken language stimulation relies on two options: (1) to present information through audition alone, or (2) to present the auditory target with visual support through speechreading (also called lipreading). Either choice can be correct depending on your objective. Some children do better if new objectives are presented auditorily only. Some need additional speechreading cues. In some instances you may do both in one lesson. For example, Molly has minimal hearing in the high frequencies. You may decide to present vowel sounds auditorily but provide extra speechreading cues for high-frequency consonants. You need to know the best mode to choose for each individual child.

Nonauditory Cues

Children can be tricky. They may rely on vision and are not truly listening but instead are watching you like a hawk. Little Brandon sees you glance down at the ball before you say, "Throw the ball." If he is not sure what you said, he will follow your eyes. You might think that he knew the word when he was actually reading your body language.

We can give subtle cues to children through our jaw movements. For example, if you say /-o-/ (as in hot) your jaw moves down slightly and if you say /ee/ (as in meet), it doesn't. You could also be raising your eyebrows every time you make a sound, or you could be leaning toward the right object on the table. Develop a third eye and watch yourself in action. If you have any doubts, videotape yourself and see if you give anything away. Children who are developing auditory-only skills should depend on their auditory sense and should ignore other cues that you may be giving them. A child may occasionally need additional visual cues. You should always provide another opportunity for auditory-only stimulation after providing the visual cue.

Obscuring Your Lips

You can obscure your lips in either an obvious way or a subtle way. Obvious ways include the use of an embroidery hoop covered with speaker cloth, your hand, or a piece of paper. Subtle ways are more natural, such as standing beside the child or turning your head. You make the decision whether to be obvious or subtle based on your objectives and your knowledge of the child.

Premises That Drive Auditory Learning

Nevins and Chute (1996) identified eight premises that teachers should understand when engaging in auditory learning activities. Although written in reference to children with cochlear implants, the premises are also valid for any child who is developing spoken language. In the next several pages we present these premises and explain their meaning.

1. "The development of speech perception and speech production abilities is the primary goal of implantation. Therefore, meaningful speech should be used as the input for listening tasks" (p. 107).

Because the goal of auditory instruction is to develop speech perception and speech production, teachers should choose meaningful spoken language activities as sources for input. The ultimate goal is for the child to use listening as the foundation for developing perception and comprehension of speech. Don't ignore meaningful environmental sounds such as laughter from another room, but focus on spoken language input as much as possible.

2. "The goal of any listening activity includes the activation of the speech/auditory feedback loop. Therefore, listening practice should always provide an opportunity for a productive response" (p. 108).

When you are doing auditory lessons with a child of preschool age, ask the child to repeat what you say. This stimulates the feedback loop that we talk about in Chapter 6. First you say it; then you give the child the opportunity to imitate what he heard. In this way you foster the child's attempts to match his production to yours. One positive by-product of this technique is that the child begins to develop an *auditory rehearsal* strategy. This is the strategy you use when someone tells you something you need to remember, such as a phone number. As you increase the length of the stimulus you are asking the child to repeat, you are developing and expanding the child's auditory memory.

3. "There are certain cognitive and linguistic precursors that are necessary for successful auditory work" (p. 109).

The child must develop additional abilities as you ask him to begin structured listening tasks. Table 3.2 provides a list of cognitive and linguistic precursors.

Table 3.2   Cognitive and Linguistic Precursor to Language Instruction

Making choices. A child needs to learn to make choices to respond appropriately to objects during listening and language activities.

Understanding that speech has meaning. Teach the child that when you say something, he should do something. For example, present a group of objects, like balls, and have the child throw one into a bucket, but only after you say, "Ball" or "Throw." Your goal is not word recognition but the ability to wait as an indication that the child knows that speech has meaning.

Eye contact. Eye contact is an indication that the child is paying attention.

Turn taking. The child must know that there is a give-and-take in communication. He needs to learn to wait for you to say something before he responds to an activity.

Vocabulary and language. Be sure that the vocabulary and language that you are using are appropriate for the child and not too complex.

4. "Cochlear implants will likely provide all children with suprasegmental speech cues. Others may have access to segmental speech information. Regardless, the ability to benefit from the implant can be sharpened with specific listening practice" (p. 111).

The majority of children who are properly fitted with hearing aids and cochlear implants can learn to understand the patterns of sounds resulting from the suprasegmentals. But just putting a hearing aid or a cochlear implant on a child is not enough. Most children require specific listening practice to make maximum use of their hearing devices. Consider the case of Miguel. He was fitted with a cochlear implant at age five. But he was enrolled in a program that did not focus on any type of auditory stimulation. After two years in this program, Miguel could detect sounds with his cochlear implant, but he could not discriminate between long and short sounds (pattern perception). When later provided with specific listening practice, he developed strong speech perception skills. However, because of the delay in providing him this structured input he will never reach his full potential for spoken language competence.

5. "If classroom listening is one of the goals of auditory practice, it follows that the content of the auditory lesson be suggested by the child's classroom curriculum" (p. 113).

Auditory comprehension content is driven by the child's communication needs. The lessons you plan need to incorporate the vocabulary, language structures, and concepts that you are exposing the child to during the other parts of her day.

6. "Listening practice should be provided with a variety of input units: the phoneme, the word, the phrase or sentence, and connected discourse" (p. 113).

You should be working at the various levels of the *Model of Auditory, Speech, and Language Development* (Figure 1.1) at the same time. Depending on the difficulty of the listening and speaking skill, you can be working on some things at the discrimination level and others at the identification level. For example, Rebekah may be just learning to distinguish the difference between Group 3 vowels and diphthongs (described in Chapter 1), but she is also working on identification of common phrases such as, "Come here," and "Jump. Jump. Jump."

7. "There is a complex relationship between language and listening skills" (p. 115).

Learning to listen helps the child learn language. Conversely, having language skills also helps the child learn to listen. You need to nurture this reciprocal relationship. When Bruce and his teacher are discussing a trip to the aquarium, it's possible that he won't understand every word the teacher says. But his language ability will help him fill in the missing piece. For example, he might hear the teacher say, "How *mmmmm* seahorses were there?" Even though Bruce didn't hear the word *many* clearly, his understanding of language gave him all the help he needed to answer the question.

8. "Tasks at the phoneme level [that is, speech per se] should be selected by the teacher based on analysis of the speech production errors made by the child" (p. 116).

When you work on discrimination and identification skills, you can gain insight into what a child hears by what he says. If the child says, "pish" for "fish," working on the discrimination between /p/ and /f/ makes a lot of sense. Analyze the child's speech errors. Determine what sounds the child can perceive auditorily and use the auditory channel to stimulate the correct production. It may be necessary to allow the child to see the speech sound on your lips ("pish" versus "fish," for example), but try that only if the child continues to make the error after you have done auditory stimulation. After showing the information on the lips, again cover your mouth and deliver the sound auditorily.

FACTORS TO CONSIDER WHEN PLANNING LESSONS

When you plan your lessons, remember that you are stimulating spoken language growth in a systematic way. Determine your goal first, and then determine your activity. Many people start with a fun activity, such as making ice cream sundaes, and then choose vocabulary and language that support the activity. This is exactly the opposite of what you should do. Determine the vocabulary, grammar, listening, and speaking objectives *first*, and then devise an activity that will support these best. Once you have established your base of instruction, start planning what you're going to do. Some factors to consider include the age of the child, adding variety, and achieving success.

Chronological Age–Developmental Age

Make sure the activities are appropriate and interesting. Match activities to the child's cognitive abilities, not too easy and not too hard. Children who are three to five years old need a lot of stimulation. They cannot be asked to do any activity for a long period of time. Practice skills in a meaningful way to promote carryover. Repeat activities over a period of days. Children need to be communicative and to have fun.

Interests

In general, three- and four-year-olds are interested only in things they're interested in. In other words, you need to match their interest level if you want to keep their attention. Children of this age love to touch, move, make, break, and so forth. You need to know what they love to do at home and their favorite foods. Perhaps Sam is not that interested in dressing the doll and would rather ball the clothes up and throw them in a hamper instead. Meet Sam halfway and set up the activity so that Sam can put the clothes in the hamper (or any basket you can find). Your goal is to have Sam say "red shirt" and "green socks." You have accomplished this goal in a way that is meaningful and interesting to Sam.

Variety of Contexts and Activities

The child needs to practice his goals in a variety of contexts. You can practice the words *up* and *down* by picking him up and putting him on his chair, by putting things up on a shelf and down on the floor, by going up and down the slide, or by climbing up and down to get in and out of the car. Keep these goals in the forefront of your mind and practice them throughout the day. Some parts of the day you will be working in structured auditory language lessons. At other times during the day, you will be working on targets in more natural auditory language experiences. Be sure that you repeat your targets in structured and natural settings all day long. No matter what happens, if you have your objectives clearly in mind, you will be more likely to stay on target. Even if your activity fails (e.g., your ice cream sundae melts before you eat it), you will still impart appropriate language stimulation.

Challenging Yet Successful

Nothing succeeds like success. Children thrive when we organize their environment to be challenging and stimulating, while making sure the child achieves success. When you challenge a child to do an activity, be sure to think through the steps you will be following and the goals you have set for the child in case you need to break down the task for the child to achieve success. You have to think one step ahead of the child all day long. What are you going to do if Jesse gets this right? What are you going to do if she makes a mistake? You need to think about this before you start the activity.

Comprehensible Input

While the language environment needs to be challenging, the child must also understand what you are saying to him. Many mainstream preschool classrooms provide a language environment that is above the level of the child with a hearing loss. The child may not understand much of what the teacher is saying and may have difficulty engaging in most conversations and therefore feels incapable of communicating. The teacher's job in this classroom is to engage the child on his level and to present information and activities that allow the child to participate fully and successfully.

Communicative Intent

You need to set up situations in which the child has a desire to communicate. The environment needs to motivate him. Children with hearing loss may encounter times when it is uncomfortable for them to participate. The teacher must be able to set up situations where the child wants to talk. Children who are deaf or hard of hearing desire to communicate, but they may need more time to formulate their response. Be sure to provide sufficient processing time by waiting for the child to respond. Explain to the other children in the classroom that, "We wait for all our friends to think and talk."

TECHNIQUES TO USE WHEN CONDUCTING A LESSON

You have designed your lesson and thought about how you are going to integrate all the different parts. Now you are ready to teach, but first let's look at some important tips or strategies to keep in your bag of tricks.

Wait for a Response

As we described in the previous section and in Chapter 2, give the child a chance to respond. Many people are inclined to fill in silences with talking. Try to avoid doing too much talking. Everything you say should be intended to elicit a response. Try waiting longer than you normally do to see if you get a response. Children who understand turn taking know that you expect them to do something. And, if you wait long enough, usually they will. The only time you wouldn't wait is if you see the child struggling to the point of frustration. Then you would step in with a hint. In these instances, you should also teach the child self-help strategies by saying, "I don't know" or "Help me" or "What?" This scripts a response for the child for times when he doesn't know what to say. You are not forcing the child to guess, or to shut down, but are gently nudging him forward by giving him permission to ask for help.

Acoustic Highlighting

Acoustic highlighting is a term used to describe the different ways that teachers emphasize or clarify a key feature of an auditory stimulus to make the feature more salient. Your goal is to move from an environment where you provide significant highlighting to one where you offer no highlighting at all. When you introduce a new skill or when the child has trouble with a skill, acoustic highlighting provides the bridge to success. Table 3.3 presents some aspects of acoustic highlighting.

Table 3.3   Aspects of Acoustic Highlighting

Aspect	Description
Repetitions	Provide many repetitions of the stimulus, moving toward providing fewer and fewer. Once the child can respond, say the word once and wait for the child to respond.
Rate of speech	Start with a slower rate, separating the words from one another and moving toward speaking at a natural rate.
Pitch and rhythm	Provide extra suprasegmental information (as in motherese), moving toward more typical prosody.
Acoustic contrast	Stress the word or sound that you want the child to listen for so that it stands out in the sentence. "I want the RED truck." Always work toward speaking naturally.
Distance	When introducing a new skill or when the child has trouble hearing, move closer. As the child gains skill remember to practice that skill at a distance.

SOURCES: Erber and Greer (1973); Nevins and Chute (1996).

Whispering

When you whisper, the consonants come out to play! The natural voicing of vowel sounds is usually so overwhelming that the child might not be able to hear the consonants. If you want the child to hear the consonant you're working on, try whispering or speaking softly (Ling, undated). When you whisper, vowels are no longer louder than the consonants.

Singing

When you sing, the vowels come out to play! Singing elongates the vowels and is great for keying into the vowels. Singing also adds prosody, phrasing, and suprasegmentals to the words. Plus, singing is fun!

Building Bridges

In the preschool classroom where all children are deaf or hard of hearing and where the teacher is specially trained to work with children who are deaf and hard of hearing, the primary focus is on communication skill development. In the mainstream preschool, there is the expectation that children will have a larger communication repertoire to draw from than is often the case. Consequently, it is very important to build a bridge between the child's existing auditory-speech-language skills and the demands of the classroom. Review previous descriptions of acoustic highlighting, expansion, expatiation, and clarification. Draw heavily on scaffolding techniques such as using pictures, focusing on key words, and paraphrasing. Effective scaffolding means that the adult adjusts her language to the child's present level while still providing challenges for communication growth (Gibbons, 2002).

Self-Correction Techniques

Teach the child to self-correct by a system of reducing available cues. Table 3.4 identifies some commonly used self-correction techniques.

Table 3.4   Self-Correction Techniques

Explicitly telling child his error and telling him what he needs to say to fix it

Telling child his error and asking him to self-correct

Telling child the category of error made (e.g., speech versus language) and asking him to self-correct

Telling child the type of error made (e.g., noun versus verb) and asking him to self-correct

Using clarification techniques. Giving cues to self-correct, such as "Excuse me?" "Would you say that again?" "Sorry, I don't understand." "Repeat that for me." or "What did you say?"

The "Sandwich" Interaction

A special style of interaction that teachers who work with children who are deaf and hard of hearing must master is the sandwiching interaction. Sandwiching is a set of techniques to help children learn new information as it relates to old information. There are several perspectives on sandwiching based on the underlying theory and the teacher's instructional purposes. The three kinds of sandwiches include: the listening sandwich, the thinking skills sandwich, and the concept sandwich (see Table 3.5).

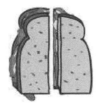
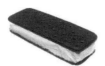

The first type of sandwich that you will use is the *listening sandwich*. This sandwich is made up of the sequence of cover-uncover-cover (described in the student examples below). We use the listening sandwich when we expect children to detect, discriminate, identify, or comprehend new or developing listening objectives. The second type of sandwich is the *thinking skills sandwich*. This is made up of the sequence of unknown-known-unknown (described in the student examples below). We use the thinking skills sandwich when we expect children to think at higher levels of cognition than are in their current repertoire. These first two types of sandwiches are based on Feuerstein's (1980) concept of Mediated Learning

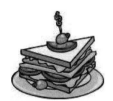

Experiences—the humanistic interactions of a teacher or mentor who selects, focuses, and organizes the array of stimuli so the child can link purposeful learning to new situations and develop self-regulated behavior (Kozulin & Rand, 2002).

The third type of sandwich is the *concept sandwich,* which follows the known-unknown-known sequence (described in the student examples below). This type of sandwich is based on Vygotsky's (1978) models of providing guidance to understand a task, process, or concept. The technique of *scaffolding* (Bruner, 1975) is also based on the work of Vygotsky. Scaffolded instruction involves teacher and peer sequencing of prompts for the purpose of providing optimal support for learning (Dickson, Chard, & Simmons, 1993). When we scaffold, we support students until they can apply new skills and strategies independently (Rosenshine & Meister, 1992).

Table 3.5   Strategy Sequences for the Sandwiching Technique

Type of Sandwich	Sequence
Listening	Cover (mouth)-Uncover-Cover
Thinking	Unknown-Known-Unknown
Concept	Known-Unknown-Known

Let's see how a teacher would use these concepts while preparing for a field trip to the aquarium. Carmen's class is getting ready to go to the aquarium. Carmen has a well-developed ability to detect sounds without much effort; she can recognize many sounds and words but not others; and she is working solidly at the identification stage. The teacher wants Carmen to listen to the names of two fish she will see on the trip. The first is a puffer, the second is an angelfish. The teacher selects the appropriate stimuli and focuses the child's attention. The teacher presents pictures of these using the cover-uncover-cover strategy, by covering her mouth as she says, "Oh look. Here's a (cover) puffer. See the (uncover) puffer? It has spots. Can you say (cover) 'puffer'?" The objective is for Carmen to demonstrate identification (brain task) of the name of a new fish (listening and speaking skill) when given the carrier phrase, "Can you say ___?" (external factor—linguistic complexity) by repeating the teacher's words (child action). The teacher repeats the same thing with the angelfish and then asks Carmen to identify the words angelfish and puffer. For example, after placing both pictures in front of Carmen, she might say, "Point to the (cover) puffer." If Carmen does not identify the fish, then the teacher would uncover her mouth and repeat the instruction.

The teacher is also working on descriptive adjectives as a target language objective. The teacher might write Carmen's objective to say: "Carmen will demonstrate identification (brain task) of descriptive adjectives (listening and speaking skill) when given a variety of pictures (external factor—closed

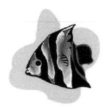

set) by choosing a picture and describing the fish (child action)." To incorporate unknown-known-unknown sandwiching into this, the teacher sets out pictures of several fish for Carmen to see. She might say, "Carmen, here is a striped (unknown) fish. It has lines (known) on it. It is striped (unknown). Here is another fish. It isn't striped. Can you show me the striped fish?"

Next, we might want to teach Carmen some new concepts. We would use known-unknown-known sandwiching to teach unfamiliar concepts. We might say: "Fish live in a giant fish tank (known). The word for this giant fish tank is 'aquarium' (unknown). It's just like the tank our guppies are in (known), only it is really, really big!" The teacher can also combine the listening sandwich with the concept sandwich, covering her mouth when she says "aquarium." Sandwiching promotes listening, language, and higher-order thinking skills, sometimes simultaneously. We could use each of the sandwiches for each of the three activities described, however, our choice of sandwich is determined by whether our focus is on listening, thinking, or concept development.

Making Progress

Sometimes after all our hard efforts, a child does not make adequate progress in his current environment. When this happens, it is important to question how well you are monitoring his overall instructional environment.

- Are his listening equipment and settings the best choice?

- Are you working at the appropriate level of brain task, or on the appropriate developmental level of speech and language objectives?

- Have you controlled adequately for external factors such as complexity of the situation in which he must respond?

- Have you made every effort to keep the family actively involved?

- Have you addressed additional needs that may stem from concomitant learning, behavior, physical, or other sensory disorders?

- Have you honestly appraised the skills of the service providers, and if they are found lacking, have you arranged for appropriate in-service instruction or collaboration from an expert?

If you can answer yes to all of these questions and the child is still not making progress in communication, then it is probably time to call the Individualized Education Program (IEP) team together to consider modifying the child's mode of communication, to involve more visual information such as speechreading, or visual communication systems (e.g., cued speech or sign language) or to consider whether he should be in a different type of classroom. We want to give a child every opportunity to learn spoken communication, but if he makes no progress after (1) extensive auditory lessons and experiences under ideal conditions, or (2) auditory lessons enhanced visually through speechreading, pictorial support, or print support, then we must consider the addition of other visual communication systems.

INTERVENTIONS FOR PRESCHOOLERS

In this section we describe the *Model of Auditory, Speech, and Language Development* (Figure 1.1) as it applies to children in the preschool years. Take advantage of the many well-organized auditory development curricula available today to plan your progression through the stages of the *Model of Auditory, Speech, and Language Development.* Some of these curricula are listed in Resource D. Following is a general description of things to think about when you plan and conduct your lessons, organized along the parameters described in Chapter 1.

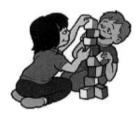

APPLYING THE *MODEL* WITH PRESCHOOLERS

Parameter 1: Brain Tasks

Brain tasks refer to detection, discrimination, identification, and comprehension. Work on these levels as described in Chapter 2 with children who are at younger listening ages.

- If the child is not at the highest levels of discrimination to beginning identification stage, he does not have the ability to learn from naturalistic interventions. Collaborate carefully with the teacher of the deaf and the speech-language pathologist on more analytic methods (Ertmer, Leonard, & Pachuilo, 2002).

- All work should be heading toward the child being able to identify and comprehend sounds of language before entering kindergarten.

- Use the technique of covering your mouth with your hand or a hoop. The point of listening activities is for the child to learn to listen. If you have given clear clues, clear speech, and a clear task objective and the child is still not able to perform the brain task you are asking for, use the concept sandwich. If the child still is unable to do the task, try it at a lower level of brain task. If he still is unable to do the task, use the auditory sandwich. If the child still has not mastered the skill, add in visual support through lipreading, print, or other means.

- Auditory brain tasks are usually the *most* overlooked component of development in the typical preschool special needs classroom. Everyone thinks to work on speech, everyone thinks to work on vocabulary, but unless you have been specially trained, you may not think to work on auditory brain tasks. The child will not make efficient progress unless you couch all your activities within the context of learning to listen.

Parameter 2: Listening and Speaking Skills

- Familiarize yourself with the acoustic characteristics of speech available to the child. You will engage in ongoing progress monitoring of the child's ability to perceive the aspects of sound that are in his range of available hearing. Build on established abilities to develop new abilities. For example, Steven may be able to tell the difference between long and short utterances, like "Hop" and "Turn around and around." You can now start to sharpen that skill by presenting him with one and two syllable words (like "car" and "popcorn").

- Minimal pairs—As you fine-tune skills with listening, you can start asking the child to choose between two words that are different in only one way. For example, these words may have the same beginning and ending consonant and only the vowel in the middle is different (*coat* and *cat*), or the vowel and final consonant are the same and the initial consonant is different (*pat* and *hat*). A child might be able to start working in minimal pairs to practice vowel and consonant identification. Be diligent that the words you use in these minimal pairs are meaningful and appropriate for the children. Minimal pair cards and word lists are available from many publishers.

- Coordinate with the other members of the IEP team on speech, language, and auditory goals. The listening and speaking goals that you pick are best supported by using the same goals in speech therapy. For example, if Anthony is working on the long /ee/ in speech class, he should practice listening to that sound during auditory lessons and auditory experiences.

- Follow a developmental curriculum to expose the child to an ever-increasing vocabulary. The average three- to four-year-old can:

  o Tell a short story of a few sentences.

  o Ask for help.

  o Answer "what," "where," and "why" questions.

  o Understand 800 to 1,500 words.

  o Use plurals, possessives, and several verb forms.

  o Follow three-step directions.

The average four to five-year-old can:

  o Use 1,000 to 2,000 words.

  o Communicate easily with a variety of individuals.

o Speak in grammatically correct sentences of eight to ten words in length, including advanced grammatical forms such as adverbial and relative clauses.

o Understand more than 2,800 words.

o Answer questions about how things function.

o Engage in complex role-playing using appropriate language

o Participate in group activities.

- Provide the child with models and practice of proper use of social language by saying, "Excuse me" if you want to move by someone, or "Help me, please" if you can't zip your jacket. Practice waiting your turn and not interrupting people who are engaged in a conversation.

- Use "mini-songs" that incorporate target vowels. See Chapter 2 for sample mini-songs.

- Begin work on combining words, phrases, and sentences. Table 3.6 identifies language and thinking skills appropriate for this age.

Table 3.6   Language and Thinking Skills That Preschoolers Are Developing

Compound Sentence Forms	• Two verbs related • Helping (auxiliary) verb and a main verb (e.g., I have eaten my peas.) • Two verbs not related (e.g., She heard the cow mooing.) • Coordinating conjunction (e.g., but, yet, so, for)
Complex Sentence Forms	• Complements (e.g., know that . . . think that . . .) • Early subordinating conjunction (e.g., because, before, after, until, when)
Thinking Skills	• Categorize serially and hierarchically • Organize events • Seriation of thoughts • Higher symbolic thought

SOURCES: Moog and Biedenstein (1999); Owens (1996); Schumaker and Sheldon (1999).

Parameter 3: External Factors

As the child becomes more mature and gains facility with listening and speaking skills, you need to add complexity to the external factors. For example, Simone is able to choose an object from a set of four objects when you say the label. You say, "Rabbit," and Simone picks up the toy rabbit. How do you make this task a little harder?

- You can add more objects to the set so that Simone is now picking from six instead of four (external factor—stimulus array).

- You could change from objects to pictures (external factor—contextual cue).

- You could embed the word in a phrase (external factor—linguistic complexity), "Pick up the rabbit."

- You could open the door to the classroom, adding background noise from the hallway (external factor—background noise).

The main point is that whenever a child is able to perform a task with relative ease, it's time for you to make it a little harder. There's no right way to make it harder. All of the above are fine. Just make it harder, one way at a time.

Parameter 4: Child Actions

Preschoolers are quite capable little individuals. They can jump, hop, walk forwards and backwards, throw a ball, build a puzzle, clap their hands, draw, color, zip, paste, copy, cut, wait, and other things that babies and toddlers can't do. The activities you choose for the child to perform to demonstrate his brain skills should be fun, age appropriate, and compelling for the child.

Derrick

Derrick is three years old. He currently has a middle ear infection in addition to his moderate hearing loss. He is in a self-contained preschool classroom for children who are deaf or hard of hearing. His class is a total communication class. The certified teacher of the deaf and hard of hearing uses sign language to support communication. Some of the students in the class depend completely on signs to communicate. Derrick can understand speech and requires sign only for clarification. Each child has a different set of goals based on his or her present levels of ability on the *Model of Auditory, Speech, and Language Development*. Derrick is able to identify words (brain task) that vary by long versus short vowel (listening and speaking skill), embedded at the end of a phrase (external factor—linguistic complexity), from an array of two (external factor—stimulus array). The children and teacher sit on the floor. The class is preparing for a trip to the aquarium, so the teacher has selected the following words: *octopus, fish, seahorse, eel*, and *crab*. The teacher talks about each of the toy animals with the children relating the objects to a book they have been reading about sea animals. The teacher pulls out the *eel* and *crab*, turns to Derrick, covers his mouth, and says, "Give me the crab." Derrick picks up the eel. The teacher says (with his mouth covered), "That's the eel. Give me the crab." The teacher employs the auditory sandwich, saying "crab" with his mouth covered, repeating "crab" allowing Derrick to see his face, and then repeating "crab" with his mouth covered again. Derrick picks up the crab and puts it in the box.

This teacher incorporated content, vocabulary, and auditory goals into one lesson. He set up an activity with appropriate materials to be flexible enough to meet each student's individual needs. He tied the activity into the real world by looking at pictures of the real animals and traveling to the aquarium.

SUMMARY

The preschool years are key years for making sure that the child with a hearing loss is able to enter kindergarten with a usable language and listening system. For the child who has had sufficient support since infancy, preschool will help round out his use of spoken language. For the child whose first school experience is preschool, the teacher's challenge is monumental. She must take a nonlistener and turn him into a listener, and she must take a noncommunicator and turn him into a communicator. This chapter recommended the following practices:

- Collaborate with a multidisciplinary team.

- Know details about the child's hearing loss, previous services, and present level of skills.

- Use the *Model of Auditory, Speech, and Language Development* (Figure 1.1) to guide you in determining appropriate goals and objectives.

- Follow the premises of auditory development.

- Incorporate all the strategies recommended where appropriate.

Interventions for Children in the Primary Grades 4

In this chapter we describe interventions for children in kindergarten and the early elementary grades. This chapter has five objectives. First we describe the effect a hearing loss will have on various aspects of school life. We review the various areas of assessment that will provide information to help determine the child's level of performance. We present the various placement options appropriate for children who are deaf or hard of hearing, describe the people who may be working with the teacher and the child, and explain the different levels of intervention necessary for a child who has developed good communication skills by kindergarten age and for a child who continues to need focused teaching to develop communication skills. The primary needs of students in the early grades include continued work on communication development, modifications to bridge the listening and language requirements of the classroom, and support in developing the ability to socialize with others.

A TYPICAL DAY IN THE LIFE OF THE YOUNG STUDENT WITH A HEARING LOSS

What is a day in the life of a deaf or hard of hearing child like when his ability to communicate and get information from his environment is affected by his hearing loss? The hearing loss not only affects his ability to hear clearly, but also disrupts vocabulary, language, and background knowledge acquisition and use.

Delays in Processing Speed

Young students who are deaf or hard of hearing experience delays in processing speed (i.e., the amount of time it takes to integrate various pieces of information). They must expend extra energy understanding what is being said, eliminating possible meanings, and deducing others because of their limited vocabulary and background knowledge. Because they have to fill in the gaps, they focus their attention on this process and may not benefit from higher-order discussions about the topic of conversation. They constantly try to play catch-up, which can be confusing, frustrating, and exhausting. Box 4.1 provides a scenario that puts *you* in the same position.

Box 4.1   Processing Speed Scenario

You are in a meeting with your boss and coworkers. Your boss hands you the following list and asks everyone to identify the items that are most fungible: tobit, eigenvectors, smoothers, cointegration, strips, heckit, arbitrage, tranversals, mantissa, polity, and bimetallists. Your boss also says that the amount of your next raise in salary will be determined by how well you respond. Your coworkers raise their hands and call out some of the items from the list that seem most fungible to them. Unfortunately for you, you don't know what fungible means and you are familiar with only five words on this list. You're not even sure if the definitions that you know of those five words are the same as the definitions everyone else is using. In addition, your coworkers are whispering their comments and you have to really strain to tell exactly what they were saying. To make matters worse, each time someone speaks, you aren't sure who is talking and have to scan the faces around the table to see whose lips are moving. By the time you figure out who is talking, you missed the beginning of what that person was saying, and now you have forgotten the definitions you had figured out. The meeting adjourns with the boss looking sharply your way, and saying, "Tsk, tsk."

Reading and Content Area Delays

Children who have significant communication delays will also have significant reading delays. When a child is presented with a written test, what may appear like a simple question may in fact be beyond the child's reach. Often even the definitions in the dictionary don't help, because he doesn't understand them either. Children who go through their days feeling helpless either start acting helpless, or they start engaging in behaviors to entertain themselves. Many children with hearing loss are mislabeled as having a behavior disorder simply because they are bored and frustrated. The child could benefit from some help breaking down the task into units that he can understand and process. This strategy will teach him problem-solving skills and give him a sense that he can master what seems insurmountable. Box 4.2 provides a scenario that puts you in the same position.

Social Interaction Challenges

Whoever said that students with disabilities belong in the regular classroom if for no other reason than for socialization completely missed a fundamental requirement of socialization: students need a communication system to allow them to socialize with each other. When thrust into a classroom of running, laughing, giggling kids who are chattering away, the child without a communication system is unable to interact and socialize, and is often the brunt of

Box 4.2   Reading and Content Area Challenge Scenario

You go back to your office and open your e-mail. You have received an e-mail that requires a response within 20 minutes. You read through the message, grabbing your dictionary so that you can look up the words you're not sure of as you go along. Here's what your e-mail says: *Please perform a generalized Weiner process calculation on the statistics you have collected.* You consult your dictionary and don't understand the definition. You ask the guy in the next cubicle how to do this calculation. He is busy and answers you quite rapidly, but you miss it. You have five minutes left to respond but you are no closer to understanding what you read than when you started. Oops, your time is up. You have failed at another task.

---

ridicule. Delays in language result in delays in socialization. Placing the languageless child in a typical classroom is like dropping him into the middle of a foreign country. Box 4.3 provides a scenario that puts *you* in the situation of social isolation.

Box 4.3   Social Isolation Scenario

You go into the employee lounge and sit with your coworkers. They're talking about something and laughing, but you can't understand exactly what they're saying because many of them are whispering again. They're eating and drinking, so their mouths are covered by their hands most of the time and you cannot read their lips. One of the coworkers turns to you and says, "What do you think about that?" You say, "About what?" Your coworker rolls her eyes and says, "Never mind. You never listen to what we're saying." You try to make a joke about yourself and say, "I'm sorry. I was up late last night. Look at me! I'm tired and *dis-hee-vuled*." Your coworkers snicker, turn their backs, and talk amongst themselves. No one ever told you how to pronounce the word *disheveled (di-shev-uled)*. It's 10:15 a.m. and you still have seven more hours of this before you can go home to catch up on the tasks you missed during the day in addition to the after-hours work your boss regularly assigns.

THE EFFECTS OF HEARING LOSS IN THE CLASSROOM

The teacher, parents, and support team (i.e., resource room teacher, speech-language pathologist, teacher of the deaf, related service providers, etc.) need to explore the effect that the regular classroom environment has on the child's speech perception and production, spoken language, vocabulary, background knowledge, peer relationships, self-esteem, and academics. In the next section, we discuss the effect a hearing loss has on each of these.

Understanding What the Teacher Is Saying

A child with a hearing loss may have difficulty understanding what others are saying and making herself understood (Alegria & Lechat, 2005). Few classrooms sufficiently modify the acoustic environment to meet the needs of the child with a hearing loss. The child may rely more on her vision in noisy situations or may hear only part of a message. Often the child will guess her appropriate response in a situation, and sometimes this guess will be wrong. A sensitive teacher will adjust situations to provide the child with as much information as possible without calling attention to the child's needs or differences. The teacher will work with the school audiologist to help determine the accommodations necessary to provide an appropriate auditory environment for the child.

Speech Production

The child with a hearing loss may have speech production problems that include misarticulating sounds, omitting sounds, and mispronouncing words (Peng, Spencer, & Tomblin, 2004). In some cases the child's peers will not have the maturity or skills to maintain the conversation and attempt to understand what the child is saying. The teacher needs to be aware of any difficulties, and then practice some strategies for working through any misunderstandings. The entire team (teachers, speech-language pathologist, and parents) need to work together on communication objectives and strategies.

Spoken Language

A child with a hearing loss may have language delays, ranging from mild to very significant. Language differences will be apparent in his understanding (receptive language) and in his use (expressive language) of language. The classroom teacher must work closely with the team and the child's parents to understand the areas of language where the child has needs in addition to his language goals.

Vocabulary

Almost all children with hearing loss have vocabulary deficits, especially as they grow older (Prezbindowski & Lederberg, 2003). As a teacher prepares a lesson, the teacher reviews the important vocabulary necessary to convey the concept. A teacher can often be caught off guard by a vocabulary word that the child with a hearing loss does not know, or a word for which the child has only minimal understanding. For example, while planning a lesson on how the earth revolves around the sun, a teacher might decide to define "revolution" as one "turn of the earth." If a child with a hearing loss only understands "turn" to mean "one after another" (as in, "my turn"), the lesson will be very confusing to the child. The teacher needs to be sensitive to possible misunderstandings brought on by vocabulary deficits. The teacher can work with the speech-language pathologist, teacher of the deaf and hard of hearing, and the child's parents to provide vocabulary words that the child can practice in therapy and individual sessions, and at home.

Figure 4.1 Child Walks Around Chair to Experience the Concept of a "Revolution"

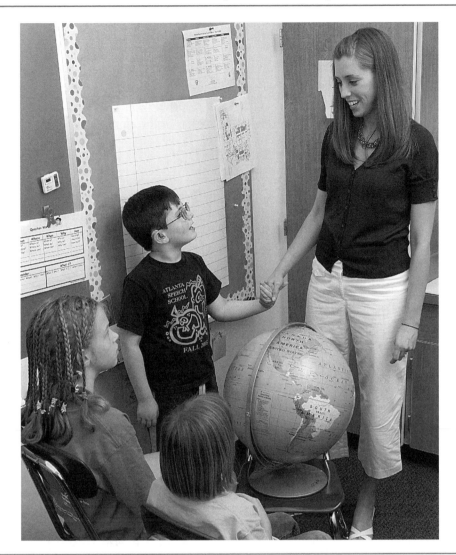

SOURCE: Photographed by John Zimmermann.

Background Knowledge

Most children with a hearing loss haven't had the same level of experience with the world as have children with normal hearing (Loeterman, Paul, & Donahue, 2002). The child who is deaf or hard of hearing tends not to learn language or acquire information through *incidental learning experiences* (i.e., to overhear and learn "through auditory osmosis"). This leaves a significant gap in his awareness of common, everyday knowledge. The child with a hearing loss may not have the same level of exposure to many cultural aspects of the community, including nursery rhymes and famous people. The classroom teacher should remain alert for instances in which a lack of fundamental understanding is leading to confusion.

Processing Speed

A limited vocabulary, problems hearing or understanding what others are saying, and unfamiliarity with the topic all contribute to a child's delay in processing the information that is presented in the regular classroom (Clark, 1991). The teacher can help by repeating the information presented, writing items on the board, encouraging the child with a hearing loss to ask for clarification, and giving the child with a hearing loss more time to answer when called upon. Prior to the lesson, the teacher should send information about upcoming topics, concepts, and vocabulary to the speech-language pathologist, the teacher of the deaf and hard of hearing, and the child's parents so that the child can preview these and participate more fully in the lesson in the classroom.

Written Language

The child will have similar needs in the area of written language as she has in spoken language (Yoshinaga-Itano & Downey, 1996). These needs can be shared and worked on with the speech-language pathologist and the child's parents. The child will need specific instruction in all aspects of writing, from style and content to grammar and usage. The teacher of the deaf and the child's parents can be a good source of support for assistance with written language. Correction of syntactical and style errors can become a natural part of the editing process that all of the children work through. Be sure there is sufficient collaboration among team members so that everyone is clear on who is providing direct instruction and who is providing remedial support.

Reading

Reading involves decoding and comprehension. We discuss reading extensively in Chapter 5. A child with a hearing loss may need specific teaching in phonological awareness and phonics to learn to decode words, along with instruction in all aspects of reading. All of the problems with comprehension brought on by language and vocabulary delays significantly affect the child's ability to understand what he is reading. Another area of weakness that appears during reading is the background knowledge the child brings to the task. The classroom teacher will work closely with the resource teacher, teacher of the deaf, speech-language pathologist, and the child's parents to be sure that the child has the decoding skills, vocabulary and language comprehension, and understanding of the necessary background information to be able to understand the information he is reading.

Math

Although many aspects of mathematics are concrete and visible, the ability to talk about how problems are solved and to relate mathematical principles to daily life requires a high level of language ability and thinking skill (Kelly, Lang, & Pagliaro, 2003). The teacher must be sure the child with a hearing loss has the vocabulary and language ability necessary to understand and explain the "why and how" of mathematical concepts. This also may require the help of the support team so that the child may practice using terms and concepts before applying them in the mainstream classroom.

Word problems are a bother for all children. The impact of a hearing loss on vocabulary, language, and background knowledge can overwhelm an

Figure 4.2   Word Problems Challenge Children With Hearing Loss

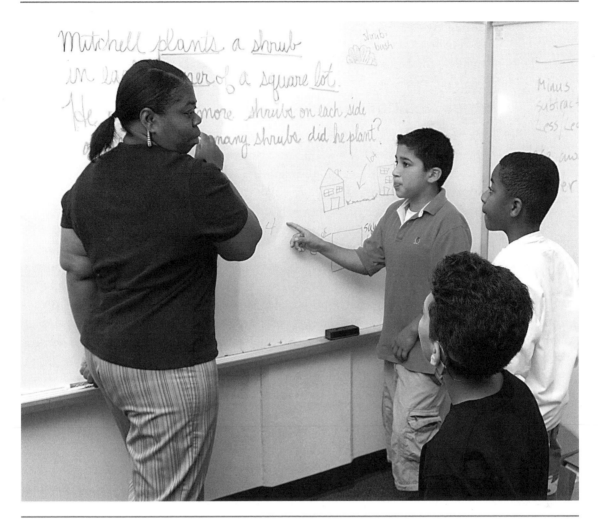

SOURCE: Photographed by John Zimmermann.

otherwise easy problem for a child. Consider the following word problem: *A pilot took a journey of three hours. The total distance traveled was 2,100 kilometers. What was his rate of speed?* If the child doesn't know what a "pilot" is and has never heard the word "journey," then he is going to be discouraged before he even begins the process of differentiating important information from unimportant information or applying the appropriate math operations. A teacher must prevent possible breakdowns and provide the child with appropriate vocabulary support.

Science and Social Studies

Consider the cumulative effects of delays in language, vocabulary, and reading. Add the extra stress of the dependence on listening that is necessary in the classroom. Now factor in that most science and social studies lessons incorporate group discussions in the class. Also add the effects of delays in processing speed that we described earlier, and you begin to get a sense of the difficulty that many elementary-age children have with social studies and science lessons (Lang & Albertini, 2001). As with math, concept development in all academic subjects is a challenge for children with hearing loss. Ask for support from the resource team to help preteach vocabulary and concepts, to develop visual organizers for information, and for instructional materials that make concepts visually clear.

Peer Relationships

Humans are social creatures. We enjoy sharing time together and develop much of our sense of self-worth from personal and social interconnections. The unwritten rules of social interaction can be difficult to discern (Kluwin, Stinson, & Colarossi, 2002). A child with a hearing loss may not perceive another's tone of voice, or may misunderstand a figure of speech and miss the subtle cues that another child would easily grasp. Routinely, a child with a hearing loss may not hear another child when that child says something to him. The child attempting to initiate conversation will soon become complacent and will find another playmate who understands more readily, leaving the child with the hearing loss alone. Ask the teacher of the deaf to come to your class regularly to provide direct instruction and discussion of the "rules" of social engagement. This will be extremely beneficial for the child with a hearing loss as well as for the other children in the class.

Self-Esteem

Imagine again: You have spent the day trying to understand what the teacher is saying. You know you have a test tomorrow, but you're not sure what it's on. You understand the meaning of only three of your ten spelling words. You tried to talk with your classmates in the cafeteria at lunchtime, but it was so noisy that you couldn't hear what they said. You thought they were talking about pickles and you said you like sour ones, but it turns out they were talking about poodles. Everyone looked at you like you were really weird. Then you didn't hear the teacher say, "Line up," at the end of recess and you are not allowed go outside tomorrow. Your classmate offered to give you one of his pencils when you couldn't find yours, but you didn't hear him and then the teacher scolded you for not having a pencil. When your classmate asked you why you were so mean and didn't want his pencil, you looked at him with big brown eyes and blinked. He said, "You're rude and stupid." Unfortunately, that time you understood him perfectly.

A child with a hearing loss needs to be able to talk frankly with someone about the challenges she faces every day (Kluwin, Stinson, & Colarossi, 2002). Parents, teachers, counselors, and friends are so important to help the child talk through issues and problem-solve solutions.

Behavior

Many of the problems that a child experiences when placed in an educational situation that is too hard, too confusing, or inappropriate will manifest themselves in behavior problems. A child with a hearing loss may act out because she is confused and frustrated. She may withdraw and not participate in the class. She may appear overactive when she feels exhausted from the strains of the day and her body requires movement to stay focused. She may try to control the conversation, respond only in ways that are comfortable to her, and avoid situations in which she doesn't understand what others are saying. You will need to examine the possible underlying factors that may be contributing to classroom behaviors and try to alleviate the underlying problems before passing judgment about the child's misdeeds.

ASSESSING A CHILD'S PRESENT LEVELS OF PERFORMANCE

Instruction for a child with a hearing loss must be based on appropriate assessment. Audiological information is needed to help the multidisciplinary team make plans to modify the acoustic environment of the classroom and so you will know what the child can and cannot hear. In addition, assessment of speech, language, reading, and academic content areas should be conducted. We have listed a number of tests in Resource B.

Professionals who conduct the evaluations should be trained to administer these assessments to students with hearing loss and to interpret the results for you. Any assessment should be accompanied by a report that explains and interprets the results. If you have any questions about the results, contact the person who administered the test. It is always possible that the results need to be examined further and that additional testing may be necessary.

Someone must take on the role of the "case manager," assimilating information from all the different evaluations. Insights from one area can shed light on another. For example, you may see that your child has a low score on a visual motor integration (eye-hand coordination) test. This could explain why she scored so poorly on the achievement tests that required her to fill in a bubble on an answer sheet. In this case, the score she received on her achievement test was not a "true" (or valid) score because it was negatively influenced by a deficit in another area. You could make a case for allowing this student more time, or giving her the test with no time limit. You could also allow her to mark her answers in the test booklet instead of using the bubble sheet. If you are diligent in evaluating all the assessments you receive, you will gain valuable information that will help you to provide your child with the most appropriate education and experience. Remember also that any assessment is merely a "snapshot" of how a child performed at a particular moment on a particular day. Your daily interactions with the child, in conjunction with and in comparison to the evaluations, provide important information that you need to share with others. Use this information wisely to prepare your lessons and plan the child's program.

Language and Vocabulary Assessments

The speech-language pathologist or teacher of the deaf can administer tests that evaluate the child's knowledge and use of various aspects of syntax, morphology, and pragmatics. There are also specific tests of semantics or vocabulary. You should receive information containing *norm-referenced scores* for receptive language, expressive language, total language, receptive vocabulary, and expressive vocabulary. Norm-referenced tests have been standardized on a large group of children and allow us to make comparisons to that group. You also may receive information containing *criterion-referenced testing* for language. Criterion-referenced testing identifies specific content the child must master to reach an acceptable level of performance and allows us to make comparisons to the curriculum. You should ask for assessments that analyze the elements of language with which the child is competent and those areas of need that require further therapy and support for development.

Speech Assessments

The speech-language pathologist (SLP) will also evaluate the child's speech production and some of the aspects of phonology. The SLP will ask the child to say various syllables or words and evaluate the "correctness" of what the child says. An SLP is trained to listen and compare all aspects of speech to a criterion of correct production. The SLP will comment on the child's voice quality. Does the child's voice sound like a typical child's should at that age? Is it too high-pitched, strained, or too nasal? The SLP will comment on fluency, or the relative ease with which the child talks. Does the child stutter or stammer? The SLP will also perform an *oral-motor exam.* In this exam, the SLP asks the child to do some movements incorporating his tongue, lips, teeth, cheeks, soft palate, and jaw. These movements are checked to see if the child has any weakness or coordination problems with the muscles and structures of the mouth that would influence the child's ability to produce the speech sounds correctly. The SLP will also do an *articulation* test. In this test the SLP asks the child to say a group of syllables or words that contain all the sounds of English. The SLP makes a judgment about how correctly the child produced the sound. Sometimes the SLP marks whether the error was an omission (the child did not say the sound at all), a substitution (the child substituted one sound for another; for example the child said "pish" instead of "fish"), or a distortion (the child said a sound that was not the correct speech sound and did not sound like another sound). The SLP will list which sounds were produced incorrectly and make suggestions for follow-up therapy.

Auditory Assessments

In addition to the audiological testing that we discussed in Chapter 1, you may receive information from testing by either an SLP or a psychologist regarding auditory comprehension of information, such as understanding of key words in a sentence. Some tests use recorded materials and the examiner may choose to use the recording or to present the test items via live voice. This will be noted in the report. The report will outline any areas of relative strength or weakness in the child's auditory ability.

Reading and Achievement

These tests may be administered by a teacher or a psychologist. Some of these tests are given to a group of children and some of them are individually

Figure 4.3   Student Participating in an Assessment

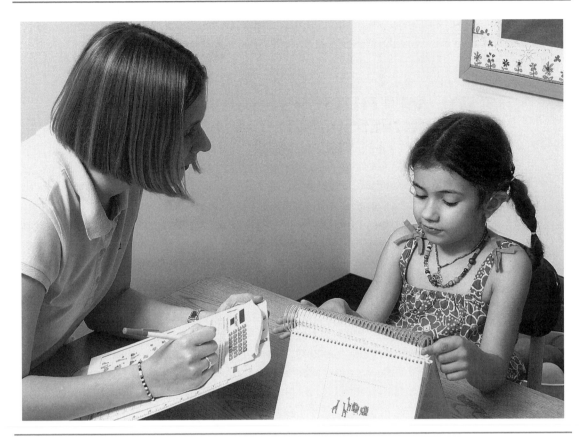

SOURCE: Photographed by John Zimmermann.

administered. Reading tests can look at various aspects of reading such as fluency, phonological processing, phonics, and comprehension. Achievement tests evaluate the child's knowledge and skill in various subjects such as math, science, and social studies. The report you will get may contain information about the areas of need in these various subjects.

Psychological and Developmental

This testing is administered by a psychologist. Usually developmental testing is done on younger children (under the age of three), and psychological testing is done on older kids. Developmental testing looks at the developmental milestones the child has achieved and usually incorporates information from the parents and teachers. Some aspects of psychological testing include intelligence, visual and auditory processing, memory, social adjustment, and visual-motor integration. The report should include areas of relative strength and weakness and suggestions of strategies for intervention.

Occupational Therapy and Physical Therapy

Sometimes an occupational therapist or physical therapist will evaluate the child. These evaluations examine the child's fine motor (small muscles) and gross motor (large muscles) abilities, balance, and the child's ability to respond to input from her senses (sensory integration). If the examiner sees any areas of need, he will recommend additional therapy and make suggestions for activities that you can incorporate in the classroom and at home.

THE MULTIDISCIPLINARY TEAM OF PROFESSIONALS WHO CAN ASSIST THE TEACHER

The team needs many individuals to help develop and provide the most effective program for a child who is deaf or hard of hearing. There is too much to learn in too short an amount of time for you to try to master everything. Use your resources. That's why schools hire teachers of the deaf, speech-language pathologists, and others. You cannot be expected to become an expert in all things pertaining to deafness overnight, which is what you would need to do to correctly serve a child with a hearing loss. Be sure that you call together a multidisciplinary team to develop an Individualized Education Plan (IEP) that will help *you.* Developing an IEP is actually a process that involves a meeting and a document. During the IEP meeting, teachers, parents, and school staff members determine the child's most effective educational program. The IEP itself is a document where all the decisions from the meeting are written down. This includes:

Needs and Goals

- Extent of involvement in the general curriculum and statewide assessments

- Services needed to achieve the goals and who will provide them

If the IEP does not help you understand how to serve the child, then it is a worthless piece of paper. Call for a new team meeting. Meet in the hallways with other service providers. Call people on the phone. Look on Web sites such as www.deafed.net, for resources where you can "Ask the Experts." Do not attempt to do this alone. Table 4.1 lists the professionals you should be courting to assist you with your deaf or hard of hearing student.

Not only is it important for a team to have a variety of members, it is also important that each member has had appropriate training in the characteristics and needs of children with hearing loss and who are learning spoken language. In order for the team truly to be multidisciplinary, more than one individual needs information expressly related to deafness (Easterbrooks & Baker-Hawkins, 1995). A professional without specific knowledge of hearing loss may have limited or inappropriate expectations. For example, some traditional practices in speech pathology will lead to a nasalized voice. The typically trained speech-language pathologist may be unaware of specialized techniques to prevent nasalization in children with hearing losses.

Table 4.1   Multidisciplinary Team Members for Students With Hearing Loss

Team Member's Title	Team Member's Job
Parents/Guardians/Caregivers	The parents provide valuable insight into the child and essential carryover of skills developed in the classroom into the child's daily life. Parents are the leaders of the support team and are to be respected and treated as such by other members of the team.
Classroom Teacher	This is either the mainstream classroom teacher or, in the case of a child who is being served in a self-contained class for the deaf or hard of hearing, a certified teacher of the deaf and hard of hearing.
Speech-Language Pathologist (SLP)	The speech-language pathologist assesses the child and provides speech and language therapy. Sometimes an SLP will also provide auditory training. The SLP can provide service to the child in the classroom and/or take the child out of the classroom for individual therapy.
Itinerant Teacher	The itinerant teacher is a teacher of the deaf who works with children placed in regular classrooms. The itinerant teacher supports the language and auditory development and academic needs of the child. The itinerant teacher may either join the child in the classroom to facilitate inclusion or take the child out of the class for individual or small group lessons. The itinerant teacher also serves as resource for the classroom teacher. Some teachers of the deaf provide auditory training.
Resource Teacher	The resource teacher is not a teacher of the deaf and hard of hearing, but may be trained in special aspects of education such as reading. The child leaves the regular classroom to spend time in the resource room with the resource teacher working on specific areas of need.
Paraprofessional	The paraprofessional (or assistant teacher) will work with the classroom teacher to support the child's interaction in the classroom.
Audiologist	The audiologist evaluates and makes recommendations about the child's hearing levels, the devices he wears, the acoustics of the classroom, and assistive listening devices. Some school audiologists also provide auditory training.
Interpreter/Captioner/Transliterator	An interpreter or captioner allows the child access to the information being presented in the classroom by either interpreting what is said or, in the case of the captioner, transcribing what is said into a computer to be read by the student. Interpreters can either be signing, oral, or cued speech transliterators.

(Continued)

Table 4.1 (Continued)

Team Member's Title	Team Member's Job
Occupational Therapist	The occupational therapist evaluates and provides therapy for the child in the areas of fine-motor coordination (including handwriting), strength, balance, and sensory-motor integration.
Physical Therapist	The physical therapist evaluates and provides therapy for the child in the areas of gross-motor coordination, strength, balance, and mobility.
Psychologist	The psychologist evaluates the child's learning style and describes strengths and weakness in the child's learning profile. The psychologist may also provide counseling.
Tutor	Tutors help children before or after school to keep up with the content of the classroom and ensure the concepts are being learned.
Counselor	The counselor meets individually or in small groups with children to discuss problems and coping strategies.

READINESS FOR SCHOOL

Children enter kindergarten and early elementary grades with an enormous range of abilities. You must have different expectations for different children. One child will not benefit from the same modifications that are appropriate for another child.

The Prepared Young School-Goer: "I'm Ready!"

Many children who are deaf or hard of hearing enter kindergarten and the early elementary classrooms with speech and language abilities in the average range. Many of these children also have average academic abilities. When this is the case, you might think that this child needs no extra support to be successful in a regular classroom, but this may be an inaccurate assumption. Even with appropriately fitted listening devices, a child with a hearing loss does not have normal hearing. The negative influence of noise in the classroom and the diminished ability for the child to acquire information through "auditory osmosis" will affect his progress. Even with superior early intervention, he must still deal with issues of language, processing time, and social frustration. These children continue to need monitoring by a speech-language pathologist and a teacher of the deaf and hard of hearing to be sure that the higher-level language structures typically acquired in the kindergarten and early elementary years do indeed develop. These higher-level skills and structures include: advanced verb tenses (e.g., present perfect: *I have taken that class.*); clauses (e.g., *unless, since, however*); questions (e.g., negative tag questions: *You would tell me if you didn't understand, wouldn't you?*); and pronouns (e.g., to represent an entire idea: *The class decided to go outside for recess. It's a great idea!).* Proper understanding and use of these structures may not develop without careful planning and stimulation from people in the child's environment. Young children with this level of skill are also ready to be challenged with tasks requiring higher-order thinking skills such as comparing and contrasting or analyzing and synthesizing.

The Unprepared Young School-Goer: "Help Me Get Started!"

A child who does not have communication abilities commensurate with his age-mates will suffer in an academically focused environment without a considerable amount of support. For a child with a significant language delay, the teacher must continue to work on communication in the context of academic concepts. The teacher must address language, speech, and auditory goals in the classroom and throughout the child's school day. The teacher must first do whatever is necessary to get the academic concept across (charts, examples, standing on her head, etc.). Next she must spend the time necessary to allow the child to practice talking about the concept, and using the language, speech, and auditory goals that are appropriate for that child.

It is not enough for a child to superficially understand a concept if the child cannot talk about it, examine it, explain it, and otherwise think about it from multiple vantage points. Few primary-grade teachers have been given the training or have the experience in continuing the process of communication development. They may have expertise in English Language Arts, but this is not language, per se. The typical primary grades classroom is driven by states' standards and curricular objectives resulting in a shift in the teaching paradigm. The primary grades teacher teaches academics rather than preacademics or developmental skills and also teaches to the "average" child, rather than the special child, whereas preschool and early intervention programs focused on optimizing communication and language development. When communication and language development have not been optimized, the child cannot benefit from traditional instruction. The IEP team should consider all options to support the child's mastery over communication while being exposed to grade-appropriate content.

INSTRUCTIONAL CONSIDERATIONS

When preparing instruction for children who are deaf and hard of hearing, teachers must consider both planning and placement.

Lesson Planning

In order to plan lessons to account for the gap between the language the child possesses and the linguistic demands of the lesson and its instruction, the teachers and therapists need to carefully collaborate. They must share and carefully discuss goals and objectives. They must carefully plan alternatives for support. The teacher's lesson plans should include a section for language, speech, and auditory goals in addition to the concepts that are being taught.

The teacher may find that the focus of part or all of one session will be on developing the concept and that subsequent sessions will require follow-up and practice with the language, speech, and auditory goals. An inclusion teacher or a paraprofessional may be involved with follow-up lessons. Every lesson developed by the teacher in collaboration with the speech and language pathologist and teacher of the deaf should include four layers of planning:

- Concept planning
- Language goals planning
- Speech goals planning
- Auditory goals planning

Table 4.2 provides a framework for planning in the areas above. Box 4.4 provides an example of how a teacher considered the four layers of planning.

Box 4.4   Sample of Planning Considerations

Mr. Jensen's first-grade class is working on a unit on plants, in particular, the concept that plants need water, sunlight, warmth, and soil. The language goals on Fredda's IEP include the infinitive (uninflected verb form: to _____; for example, *to eat*), pronouns *we* and *they,* and the conjunctions *before* and *after.* Her speech goals include the production of the /s/ sound in the final position in words and the -ee-. Fredda's auditory goal is that she will demonstrate identification and comprehension (brain tasks) of -ee- versus -o- (listening and speaking skill) given words and in phrases of four words in length (linguistic complexity—external factor) by repeating the phrases correctly (child action). Mr. Jenson collaborates with Mrs. Troutman, the teacher of the deaf, and Ms. Gilbert, the speech-language pathologist. The collaborative notes from the team meeting indicate the following:

Concept: Plants need water, sunlight, warmth, and soil.

Language: Infinitive: Plants need to have water. We have to put plants in the sun.

Plants need warmth to grow.

Pronoun: Plants are living things. They need water to live.

Conjunction: You need to water your plants after you put them in the soil.

Speech: /s/: plants, pots; -ee-: need, seed, we

Auditory: -ee- versus -o-: seed, need, we versus pot, hot, lot (e.g., a lot of water!)

They also determine who is responsible for each aspect of the unit and how tasks will be accomplished. For example, Mrs. Troutman, the teacher of the deaf, might work on teaching about infinitives and their uses. She might also work on listening activities by comparing the sounds identified. Ms. Gilbert, the SLP, might work on teaching the child to say the correct sounds. Mr. Jensen would focus on incorporating language, speech, and auditory goals into the lesson to reinforce what the others have worked on. For example, when the child mispronounces the word "seed," he could ask her to repeat the word "the way you do for Ms. Gilbert." He might also provide Fredda with auditory experiences including asking her to "plant the seed" or "pull the weed." Later he will engage Fredda in a conversation about the garden he is planting to help her extend her ability to listen to and use the words and language structures she is practicing.

Table 4.2   Collaborative Lesson Plan Form

Language Goals: _____

_____

_____

_____

_____

_____

_____

Auditory Goals: _____

_____

_____

_____

_____

_____

Concepts:

_____

_____

_____

_____

Speech Goals: _____

_____

_____

_____

_____

_____

_____

Vocabulary: _____

_____

_____

_____

_____

_____

_____

Placement Options

A child with significant delays in language development will continue to need the support of individuals addressing ongoing communication development all through the elementary years. The appropriate range of placement options must be made available to each child with a hearing loss, and placement decisions must be made with consideration of the child's communication needs. A placement is appropriate only if it is working for the child on all levels, including academics, communication, social, emotional, and physical. Table 4.3 briefly explains the different placement options that the IEP should consider.

Each one of these placements is appropriate depending on the needs of the child. Children learn and grow, and needs change over time. The support team must continually examine the child's academic, linguistic, physical, social, and emotional development, and monitor progress to verify that the placement remains appropriate for the child. If there are indications that it is not, then all alternatives should be reconsidered.

Table 4.3   Placement Options That IEP Teams Should Consider

Placement	Description
Full inclusion with or without consultative services	No special supports provided. The child is perfectly successful in a regular classroom, making adequate academic progress, continuing to develop language mastery, and making friends with his peers. This student's teacher may receive consultative services from a specialist periodically.
Full inclusion with a 504 Plan	The child is making adequate progress with the help of assistive listening devices and/or other technology.
Full inclusion with in-class support	The child is making adequate progress with the help from an inclusion teacher or a coteacher in the classroom who facilitates academic, language, and social development.
Partial mainstreaming with pull-out support	The child is making adequate progress with the help from the support team, usually with the teacher of the deaf, who is taking the child out of the classroom for individual or small-group sessions.
Resource room or self-contained deaf and hard of hearing classroom with partial mainstreaming	The child is making adequate progress spending most of the time in a smaller classroom with a teacher of the deaf and other members of the support team and going into the regular classroom for some parts of the academic day. Sometimes a member of the support team will go with the child into the mainstream classroom to facilitate inclusion.
Resource room or self-contained deaf and hard of hearing classroom with mainstream for enrichment (art, music, etc.)	The child is making adequate progress spending all of the time in a smaller classroom with a teacher of the deaf or other members of the support team and going into the regular classroom only for enrichment activities.

Placement	Description
Resource room or self-contained deaf and hard of hearing classroom with no mainstreaming	The child is making adequate progress spending all of the time in a smaller classroom and enrichment activities with a teacher of the deaf and members of the support team.
Self-contained day class in a school for the deaf	The child is making adequate progress spending all of the time in a school for the deaf. This placement would be in a school that did not have any students with normal hearing. The peer group for students in this placement would all be deaf or hard of hearing.
Residential school for the deaf	The child is making adequate progress spending all of the time in a school for the deaf. The child lives at the school.

INTERVENTIONS FOR CHILDREN IN THE PRIMARY GRADES

Let's look at some general helpful advice for a teacher who has a child with a hearing loss in the class. We'll call this child, William. When talking to William, you must pay close attention so you know when he has understood conversation and when he has not. Sometimes words sound the same or look similar on the lips. For example, some kids might ask William, "Where are you going?" and he might think they asked, "When are you going?" Obviously if William misunderstands the question, because of mistaking "when" for "where," his answer will be inappropriate and may cause others to laugh. William may be embarrassed when he discovers his error. When the time seems right, try to let William in on the joke and encourage him to ask you to repeat or to let you know when he has not understood. However, sometimes misunderstandings occur and neither the speaker nor William realizes that there has been a misunderstanding. When in doubt, check to see if William misunderstood and make an effort to clarify. Box 4.5 presents specific strategies the teacher can use to help William deal with communication breakdowns. The teacher will also need to make some modifications to facilitate the language of instruction in the classroom. Box 4.6 suggests strategies in this area. Box 4.7 provides suggestions for supporting academic instruction.

Box 4.5   Tips for Handling Communication Breakdown

Signal to teacher. Develop ways the child can acknowledge confusion without drawing attention to him.

Repeat. When the child doesn't understand you, repeat once, perhaps slowing down a bit, using *clear speech* (www.oticonus.com has a downloadable brochure about Clear Speech) and emphasizing key words or phrases. It's OK to talk to him about the concept of clear speech so he can use this as a tool to correct himself.

Simplify. Repeat your meaning, but use fewer words.

Rephrase. Try to rephrase what you have said, speaking in shorter, simpler sentences and using words that are better identified by context, are simpler, or are easier to lipread.

(Continued)

(Continued)

Elaborate. Give the child more information and build from what he already knows.

Substitute. If a word is not in the child's vocabulary, repetition will not help. Use a more common word or a word that is easier to lipread. After you have communicated the idea to him, you can repeat the unknown word for him as a way to increase his vocabulary.

Pair. Compare a known word (either same or opposite meaning) with the misunderstood or unknown word.

Delimit response. Give the child response choices. This will give him a mind-set for understanding what was said.

Build from known information. Pick a key word that will cue the child to the topic or main idea and then repeat what he did not understand.

Give feedback. Provide feedback concerning portions of the message that have been understood.

Box 4.6   Tips to Facilitate Classroom Communication

Seating. Assign the child a seat near the front of the room and off to one side. Position him so that he has a view of the entire classroom. Do not, however, have him sitting so close that he has to look up constantly. Be sure to face the child when speaking, since lipreading may help him understand what is said.

Use clear speech. Speak naturally, in a clear voice.

Stress sentence phrases. Stressing the phrases of sentences when you talk makes the information more easily perceived (e.g, "Line up {pause} for the lunchroom {pause} everybody."). Do not exaggerate your lip movements and do not cover your mouth or mumble.

Be sensitive to embarrassment. Some children are embarrassed to ask for repetitions. When a child has trouble, clarify information with him when other students are not present or when they are busy with something else.

Monitor conversations with peers. Encourage the child to participate in activities and discussions with the other students, but be ready to recognize when he is having trouble. He may have difficulty comprehending the language used in discussion or in the directions of a specific task. If the child seems confused about directions, assignments, or other information, have others repeat or simplify their sentences.

Monitor group discussions. When the child is involved in a group discussion, let him know who is talking and give him time to look at the speaker. Ask all students to speak clearly, rather than single out the child with the hearing loss because everyone in the class will better understand a clearer speaker. When it is possible and convenient, rephrase the important aspects of what has been said before calling on the next person. This often helps everyone.

Sit in a circle. Sitting in a circle is particularly helpful for group discussions because it makes it possible for the child to see everyone and for everyone to see him. Seeing the child when he talks helps the listener in much the same way as seeing the speaker helps the child.

Do not emotionally load the group situation. Correct mispronunciations discreetly. This may be accomplished by a brief conference at the end of the period or day. Some teachers keep a list of words with which the student has had difficulty and then give them to the student with the correct pronunciation later.

Control classroom noise. The quieter the room, the easier it is for the child to understand conversation. The cochlear implant or hearing aid is not as good as the ear in suppressing background noise and picking out the important voice. The cochlear implant or hearing aid amplifies everything. Follow the suggestions in Chapter 6 on reducing room noise.

Lipreading or *speechreading* is easier when:

1. The child's back is to the major source of light. It is difficult to see the speaker's face when facing into bright light.
2. The speaker avoids standing in a dark area. Try to leave a light shining on your face if instructing in a darkened room.
3. The speaker does not move around while talking.
4. The speaker speaks clearly and distinctly and faces the child when talking.

Provide opportunities for positive social interactions.

Encourage the child's independence.

Box 4.7   Tips for Helping With Academics

Listening buddy. Provide a peer listening buddy to sit next to the child to make sure the child turns to the correct page, to clarify something the teacher has said, or to provide other appropriate assistance. The listening buddy may be rotated weekly or monthly, or a few classmates may volunteer for an extended period of time. Exercise caution so that the buddy provides assistance only when needed. Take care to avoid the child's becoming overly dependent on classmates.

Study guide. Providing the child with a study guide is a great help. The child will find it much easier to follow the discussion if he knows ahead of time what will be discussed in class. Also, having him read about a topic before it is discussed in class rather than after would help him participate in class.

Vocabulary list. A list of topical vocabulary with definitions will help the child. Encourage him to use the dictionary to aid in pronunciation.

Use an overhead projector or LCD projector. Overhead projectors work very well with students with a hearing loss because a teacher faces the students while communicating the important points, and the light from the projector illuminates the teacher's face, making it easier to see.

Use captioned video. Captioned video tapes make it possible for persons with hearing loss to participate more fully and have been found useful for improving reading skills in students with normal hearing. Many videos are already close captioned. Your school should have televisions that contain a decoder chip. Open captioned videos are available with no charge through the Captioned Media Program (www.cfv.org).

Monitor spoken directions during testing. Oral examinations that require written responses may cause the child considerable difficulty. If he is writing a response while you are giving another item,

(Continued)

(Continued)

he may miss several items. Projections and transparencies work well in this case. Use words in context when presenting isolated words, as in spelling lessons. You may also give spelling tests by providing the contextual words of sentences on a sheet of paper, leaving blank spaces for the spelling words. Remember, many words appear alike on the lips and may sound alike, for example, *beet* and *bead.*

Give verbal directions before handing out visual materials. If you use pictures with verbal presentations, first describe the material and then show the illustration. Give verbal directions before handing out the materials or papers. This allows the child to focus on one major stimulus at a time.

Write all assignments on the board. When presenting an assignment, especially homework, write it on the board in addition to giving it orally.

Preteach new concepts. The regular classroom teacher can work in cooperation with the resource teacher and speech-language pathologist to cover topics presented in class. The regular classroom teacher informs the resource teacher and SLP of the lessons or concepts to be taught, and they are presented first to the child in a one-to-one or small-group setting. The child then attends the regular classroom, and the regular classroom teacher teaches the unit of study. After the class, the regular classroom teacher provides feedback to the resource teacher or SLP by means of a short note.

Watch for signs of fatigue. Students with hearing loss may experience fatigue more easily than other students. Such fatigue should not be interpreted as boredom, disinterest, or lack of motivation. The fatigue results in part from the continuous strain of lipreading, the use of residual hearing, and the constant watching required to keep up with various speakers while participating in classroom activities. It may be helpful to vary the daily schedule so that the child is not required to attend to academic subjects for an extended period of time. You may shorten class periods or alternate written and oral work with rest periods. However, the child should be expected to complete all assignments.

Ease into spoken classroom participation. In class discussions, the child may choose not to talk, but instead may be a passive participant. Allow this at first, but when he appears to be ready, encourage participation. When the child has to give reports, give the other students a written copy to follow. This will make his speech easier to understand and will make the experience more successful for both the child and his listeners. Break into smaller groups for projects or group work. As the child becomes comfortable expressing himself in small groups, he may be more comfortable in the large group.

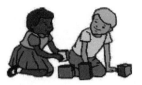

APPLYING THE *MODEL* WITH KINDERGARTNERS AND EARLY ELEMENTARY CHILDREN

Recall the *Model of Auditory, Speech, and Language Development* presented in Chapter 1 and referred to in Chapters 2 and 3. The IEP team will want to consider the child's needs relative to this model.

Parameter 1: Brain Tasks

Because children may have received anywhere from intensive services to no services whatsoever before coming to your class, there will be a wide range of abilities among children in the early elementary years. A child who has only recently begun intervention will need to start at the beginning with discrimination and identification tasks. You will also be engaging in tasks and activities associated with toddler and preschool levels (see Chapter 3). The difference is that older children may be able to do these task in the context of higher-level child actions.

Parameter 2: Listening, Speaking, and Language Skills

Work in the context of connected speech as much as possible. Children in kindergarten and early elementary school often do not receive the amount and rigor of listening and language support as do younger children. For this reason you will need to be aware of the child's speech, listening, grammar, and vocabulary goals and incorporate them into all instructional activities. You will be asking him to listen to sounds in words and key words in sentences. You will also be asking him to listen for the sounds you are learning in phonics class. Have him participate in connected discourse tracking (described in Chapter 1). Syntax and morphology objectives at this age will depend on the skills the child brings to the classroom. Children in the early elementary years typically understand even the most difficult aspects of complex grammar. If the elementary-age child does not possess the same level of skill, extra effort must be made to help him master grammar. Some grammar skills that school-age children confront on a daily basis include but are not limited to:

- Advanced tense forms such as present and past perfect tense (e.g., She had been trying for days to learn to juggle.)

- Passive voice sentences (e.g., The hunter was stalked by his own prey.)

- Dependent clauses with multiple associated independent clauses (e.g., The man, who was always late, arrived at his interview after the appointed hour but before the end of the day.)

- Indirect object location before the direct object (e.g., Jim poured his friend a Coke.)

- Sentences beginning with noun complements (e.g., That he was excited was an understatement.)

- Participial forms (e.g., Having cleaned his plate, he left the dinner table.)

The challenge to the teacher is to find appropriate ways to break these sentences into their constituent parts so that the structure does not obscure the meaning. Some suggestions follow. For advanced tense forms, make the time frame obvious (e.g., The sentence above might be rephrased: She is trying to learn to juggle. She started many days ago.). For passive voice sentences, place them in active voice order (e.g., The lion stalked the hunter.). Break sentences with multiple clauses into several separate sentences (e.g., The man was always late. He arrived before the store closed, but he missed his interview appointment.). For sentences with moved indirect objects, make the recipient of the action clear (e.g., Jim poured a Coke for his friend.). Restate sentences with noun complements more directly (e.g., He was very excited. Everyone could see.). Make the time sequence of a participial evident (First I said my goodbyes, and then I left.). Use the unknown-known-unknown sandwich (see Chapter 3) to help unveil the meaning underlying higher-level language.

Vocabulary skills are noticeably delayed in almost all young children with hearing loss (Prezbindowsi & Lederberg, 2003). Expect that you will have to provide clear explanations of commonly used vocabulary. Use clip art and Internet image searches to show pictures of vocabulary items with which the child is not familiar. Make vocabulary notebooks and share these among the teacher, speech-language pathologist, and home. Get a good vocabulary development program and continually expose the child to new words, multiple meanings, and figurative expressions. Avail yourself of several Web sites that will print out grade-appropriate vocabulary lists (e.g., www.edhelper.com/vocabulary.htm). Be relentless.

Parameter 3: External Factors

Make sure that lessons have a level of complexity that will make tasks challenging to the older child, even if you are working on simpler brain tasks or on easier listening, speaking, and language skills. Be sure to use materials that are motivating, interactive, and challenging. You may be able to ask the child to consider larger sets of stimuli. You may be able to embed the listening goal into a longer sentence. You may be able to provide fewer contextual cues. At this level you should be asking the child to make a cognitive connection. For example, you might ask, "What animal has feathers but does not fly?" instead of saying, "Point to the ostrich." Or you might ask, "What do you need to make a peanut butter and jelly sandwich?" instead of, "Show me the bread, the jelly, and the knife." Classroom noise will remain a concern.

Parameter 4: Child Actions

Expect the kindergarten- or elementary-age child to perform many different behaviors. Children can write words presented auditorily. They can do math problems on the board as the teacher reads the problem out loud. They can do connected discourse tracking or listen to a story read aloud and then tell the story back to the teacher, and/or answer questions about the story. During a geography lesson, ask them to point to states on a map as you read them aloud. For example, "Point to North Carolina and Mississippi." You could ask them to look at the map and answer the question, "Which two states border Florida?" or "Point to the state that is famous for making cheese." "Which state is called the Peach State?" Continue to make connections between curriculum goals and speech, language, and listening goals.

SUMMARY

A child with a hearing loss will need special attention in a regular classroom even if she has developed the basic skills necessary to be successful. This chapter described some of the effects of hearing loss, provided ideas for making classroom conversation more accessible, suggested modifications to bridge the listening and language requirements of the classroom, and made suggestions for support in developing the ability to socialize with others. Take advantage of the large support group that comprises the multidisciplinary team.

Some children are not ready for the communication tasks required in the regular classroom. Children with continued communication needs must be given the appropriate support. An array of appropriate placement options should be available for a child who is not being successful and communicative in the regular classroom. It is your obligation to seek out the appropriate environment when the child's placement is not promoting adequate progress.

Developing Literacy Skills in Children With Hearing Losses 5

In this chapter we will describe the process of learning to read, the factors that lead to success in reading, and the effect that a hearing loss can have on an individual's ability to learn to read. The major objective of this chapter is to describe the interdependency of spoken language and literacy in the reading development of young children who are deaf or hard of hearing.

LEARNING TO READ

The printed word is a symbol for the spoken word. Letters are symbols for speech sounds. The process of learning to read and write involves learning a printed code. Emerging readers are engaged in a process of learning to map this visual code onto the language that they have already developed.

The process of reading also involves the ability to create meaning. The eventual outcome that we are looking for when we pick up something to read is to create in our minds a thought or image from the words on the page. When we read, we are actively engaged in a complicated process involving much more than translating symbols to sounds. The goal we strive for is comprehension.

Children with normal hearing have been learning language and developing world knowledge for many years before they begin the reading task. Language and experience are not issues for them. Children with normal hearing have had experience playing with language, telling jokes, singing songs, and making rhymes. They have available skills with figurative language, inference, and multiple meanings. In the absence of a reading disability, after children with normal hearing learn to decode the words, they automatically understand what they are reading. Reading comprehension is based on background experience with the topic being read; proficiency with all aspects of language; the ability to decode the words; remembering the words while reading; and the ability to reason through any misinterpretation that is encountered (see Figure 5.1).

Now consider a young child with a hearing loss. This emergent reader may be quite different from a child with normal hearing. While a child with normal hearing comes to the reading lesson with mature and sophisticated language skills, a child with a hearing loss may come to the reading task with immature language and vocabulary. Even though the child interacts with the world around him, if nobody talks to him or he misperceives what is said, he misses out on lots of information. He may understand that a bird flies, but he may not know that some birds are called cardinals and others are called finches, that birds eat seeds and berries, or that some are migratory.

When we talk to a child about his world we call this "mediation." If the child misses out on listening to someone mediate the world for him, his world

Figure 5.1   Relationships Among Literacy Processes

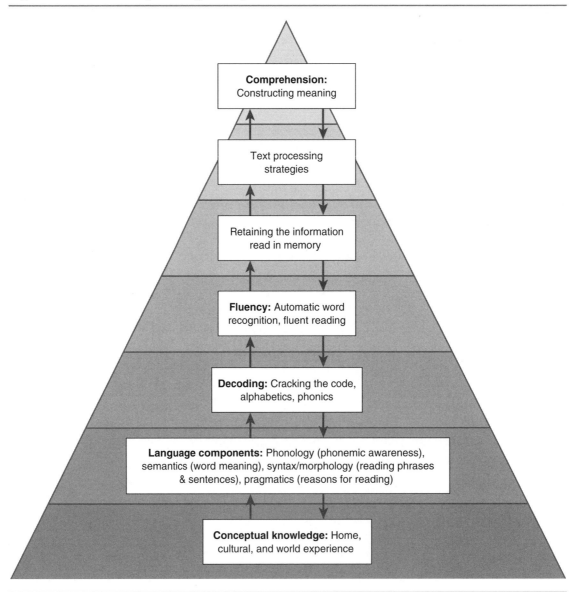

knowledge and experiences remain limited. There is an intimate synergistic relationship between thought and language. Each feeds the development of the other. This relationship is discussed further in Chapter 6. Language and experience help the child develop a bigger and bigger base of skills that support all the challenges of reading. Without this base of language and thought, the reading process is problematic. Children are asked to attach symbols to the sounds of language that may not be meaningful in their world of experiences.

Remember that the goal of reading is comprehension. It is essential during instruction for emerging readers that the child understands completely what she read. Most programs for beginning reading use vocabulary and sentence structure from the language level of a two- to three-year-old. This means that the words and sentences that children are expected to read are well within the language level of the typically developing child with normal hearing. This allows the teachers to focus on cracking the code of print without significant concern for the child's ability to understand the text. Typically developing children receive instruction in comprehension strategies after they are in the third grade, when decoding and fluency have been established. Typical reading curricula use vocabulary, language, and other terms that are often outside of the language ability of a child with a hearing loss. This child must learn what the reading process is all about before being asked to develop strategies for higher-level text comprehension. To do this, teachers must control the materials, vocabulary, and sequence of activities, making sure that they are within each child's language level.

Dianna

Establishing the Foundation

Reading Objective: Dianna will demonstrate identification of (brain task) three words that start with the /b/ sound (language and phonemic awareness task) by taking toys from a pile (child action) when the teacher labels the objects for her (linguistic complexity). The items that the teacher has selected to use are: boat, sled, plastic orange, bee, bed, drum, cup, and shoe.

Since this is a phonemic awareness lesson and not a vocabulary lesson, the teacher must be sure Dianna knows the language (vocabulary words) before she is presented with the phonemic task. If Dianna is straining to remember what the objects are, she will not be able to focus her effort on the phonemic awareness skill being developed. Before conducting the phonemic awareness activity, the teacher determines that Dianna does not know the words drum, sled, and bee. She conducts lessons providing Dianna with experience with these words and the concepts involved in interacting with them so that she is familiar with the vocabulary prior to conducting the phonemic awareness lesson. In this lesson, the teacher is reaching way down to the bottom levels of the pyramid (Figure 5.1) to teach the language and ideas that are the foundation for her phonemic awareness lesson. By learning the underlying language, Dianna can focus her energy on the reading skill that the teacher wants her to learn, identifying words by initial sound.

One of the main jobs of teachers, parents, and clinicians is to ensure that the developing reader connects meaning to reading. Ensuring comprehension requires understanding of the child's current speech perception abilities, vocabulary level, and level of language development. The teacher presents only those materials and lessons that are within the child's capability to perceive and comprehend.

In addition to having a sufficient language base in order to understand what is being read, a child must also have sufficient language and metacognitive skills

---

Dauntay

Ensuring Comprehension

Reading Objective: Dauntay will read sentences (brain task based on comprehension) fluently (child action) containing verb idioms (e.g., throw up, run on, give in; language task) in stories at his instructional reading level (external factor of linguistic complexity).

Before giving Dauntay a book to read, the teacher teaches him the concept and presents several other lessons showing him verb idioms. She uses a semantic web (see Figure 5.2), and together they build a verb idiom list. He becomes very familiar with the concept. The teacher then presents Dauntay with a book that has many verb idioms in it. As they read the book together, the teacher models fluent reading of verb idioms. Later, when Dauntay is reading a new story, he comes across the sentence, "Daddy turned on the hose, and we ran in the spray." At first he reads, Daddy-turned (pause) on-the-hose," but then he repeats himself and says, "Daddy-turned on-the hose," with a big smile on his face. He smiles because he has connected the language of the verb idiom to the print and understands the meaning of the sentence.

Figure 5.2   Dauntay's Word Web

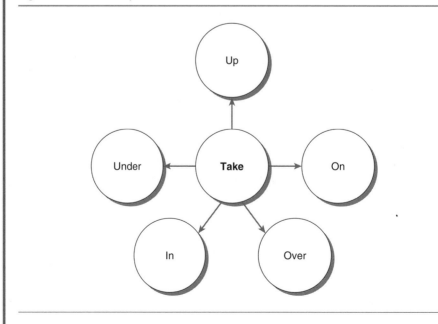

to talk about the reading process. For example, a kindergarten objective from a state department of education standard might indicate that the child "makes predictions from pictures and titles." The teacher is required to document that she has attempted to teach this lesson. Imagine what this means for Stephanie, a five-year-old who has a severe hearing loss and knows only a few words. Until Stephanie has a language base, she will not understand either the words the teacher is using or the ideas she is talking about. The most appropriate focus of Stephanie's lessons would be intensive language stimulation and development, not making predictions as part of a reading comprehension strategy.

EFFECTIVE APPROACHES TO READING

In 2000, the National Institute of Child Health and Human Development published a report that identified factors that are important in learning to read (see Table 5.1).

The next sections of this chapter will describe each of these aspects of

Table 5.1   Factors Important to Learning to Read

Alphabetics	
Phonemic Awareness	The ability to focus on and manipulate the sounds in spoken words
Phonics	A way of teaching reading that stresses the acquisition of letter-sound correspondences and their use to read and spell words (Harris & Hodges, 1995)
Fluency	The ability to read text with speed, accuracy, and proper expression. Fluency depends on well-developed word recognition skills.
Comprehension	
Vocabulary	Word knowledge
Text Comprehension	Whether the reader knows that he does not understand what he is reading, and what he does if he recognizes that he has an understanding failure

reading and examine the influence that hearing loss may have on this skill. We will review *underlying assumptions* about each aspect of reading and discuss the extent to which these assumptions are true for teaching children with hearing loss to read. Our intent in this chapter is not to provide a comprehensive reading curriculum; many of those are already available. Our intent it to identify the differences you must consider and the modifications you may need to make when using a general education curriculum with a child with a hearing loss.

Alphabetics

Alphabetics refers to a broad variety of skills associated with understanding and using letters. If young children with hearing losses are going to learn to read and write the English language, then they must understand the alphabet (Luetke-Stahlman & Nielson, 2003). The alphabet is actually two separate systems: a sound system (e.g., the sound /f/ as in *far*) and a letter name system (e.g., the name of the letter is "ef"). When children who are deaf or hard of hearing begin to read, learning the sounds of the letters is more important than learning the names of the letters. The ability to manipulate the sound-symbol relationship is called *phonics.* The literature on the subject is very clear: children with hearing losses are better readers if they are able to apply the phonics system to reading (Kelly, 1993; Leybaert, 1993, 1998; Perfetti & Sandak, 2000; Trezek & Wang, 2006).

Phonological awareness is an overarching term that describes the ability to identify, segment, blend, and otherwise manipulate the broader aspects of words and sentences. For example, a phonological awareness activity could be to count the number of words in a sentence or segment a compound word into its component words. *Phonemic awareness* is one aspect of phonological awareness that involves the manipulation of the speech sounds (phonemes) in words. For example, you might ask the child to count the number of sounds in a word, or to segment a syllable into sounds. Phonemic awareness skills are the finest distinctions that are made in the hierarchy of phonological awareness skills. Children practice phonologic and phonemic awareness skills before beginning phonics instruction, establishing an understanding of sounds in words as a foundation to learning specific letter-sound correspondences.

Underlying Assumptions About Alphabetics

The first assumption that underlies alphabetic awareness is that putting hearing aids or cochlear implants on a child with a hearing loss insures that he will be able to hear the differences among the sounds in the words. Hearing technology in and of itself will not provide access to the sounds of words; children must have extensive, systematic, and comprehensive instruction in learning to listen to sounds, as described in earlier chapters. A comprehensive listening program that prepares a young child to hear well enough through his listening devices may take many years. A young child who is not performing within six months of his normally hearing peers on tests of listening and language skills must receive specialized instruction that focuses on listening and language development.

The second assumption we must examine is that when the child decodes a word, he will understand what that word means. Decoding is a process of producing sounds associated with letters, blending the sounds, saying the word, listening to what one has just said (auditory-feedback), recognizing the word, and understanding its meaning. When a student has a hearing loss, we cannot assume that he recognizes or understands the words he is decoding. The child might be able to match a sound to a letter or letter pattern (e.g., -ing) and may even be able to sound a word out, but when you ask him what he has just read, he may not be able to tell you. Children who have hearing losses tend to come to school (whether at age three or later) with large gaps in their vocabulary.

Table 5.2   Basic Skills Associated With Print Concepts, Alphabet Recognition, Phonemic Awareness, and Phonics

---

Print Concepts

The understanding of concepts relating to the features and organization of printed text

   The ability to recognize words and word boundaries

   The ability to view text with the proper directionality (left to right; top to bottom)

   Knowledge of story grammar (beginning, middle, and end)

Alphabet Recognition Skills

The conscious awareness of letters

   The ability to recognize letter/sound (grapho-phonemic) correspondence

   The visual ability to recognize and match letters in different contexts and forms

   The ability to distinguish among the letters that are similar in appearance

   Recognition of complex orthographic elements (e.g., "ough," "ck")

Phonological Awareness Skills

The ability to focus on and manipulate words, syllables, and sounds

   The ability to segment sentences into words

   The ability to recognize and produce rhymes

   The ability to blend, segment, and delete word parts

   The ability to retrieve phonological information from long-term memory

Phonemic Awareness Skills

The ability to focus on and manipulate phonemes in spoken syllables and words

   The ability to isolate and match initial, medial, and final phonemes

   The ability to segment, isolate, and blend phonemes in spoken words

   The ability to manipulate phonemes through deletion, substitution, and shift

Phonics Skills

The conscious awareness that phonemes relate to the alphabetic system

   The ability to relate a speech sound to that sound in print

   The ability to produce a speech sound by looking at print

   The ability to segment, isolate, and blend syllables in print form

   The ability to write a letter, word, or syllable when given the spoken form

   The ability to remember sight words that contain one, two, or three syllables

---

SOURCES: Carnine, Kameenui, Silbert, and Tarver (2003); www.ed.gov/teachers/how/read/edpicks.jhtml

Decoding practice must be conducted within the context of words within the child's vocabulary. Learning to decode unknown words will not teach the child the purpose behind the decoding.

   The third assumption often made in trying to teach children with hearing loss to decode words is that the sequence we follow for children who are deaf or hard of hearing should be the same sequence we follow for children with normal hearing. In some phonics programs, work at the sound level of words proceeds from whole to part, presenting the child with a word that she does not recognize in print, then helping her analyze and synthesize the parts until she recognizes it. Some phonemic awareness and phonics programs begin with speech sounds that are difficult for the child with a hearing loss to perceive and distinguish (e.g., short vowels, high-frequency/low-intensity consonants). What is the "naturally developing sequence" for a deaf child? The professional literature is not totally clear on this, but certainly moving from largest units to smallest units when the word is not in a child's vocabulary, or working on sounds that are hard to hear will be problematic. The process must differentiate among levels of word awareness. These include:

- Providing instruction and practice with the understanding of what a "word" is

- Building up a vocabulary of meaningful words in the child's oral vocabulary

- Establishing listening skills to at least the identification level for the sounds being worked on

- Working on listening to the sounds across words (e.g., *me* versus *she*)

- Putting the sounds together by working part to whole to reveal the relationship of the sound to the word for the child

- Working in the opposite direction to take the word apart once this relationship has been revealed

- Working on onset and rime relationships once the child has a lexicon of meaningful words from which to draw

Before we move on to fluency, there is a fourth assumption to discuss. This assumption is that teaching auditory lessons based on a traditional auditory training curriculum will be sufficient to prepare the child to use phonological and phonemic awareness skills. While it is true that intensive work to develop listening skills provides children who are deaf or hard of hearing with significant precursor skills for phonological and phonemic awareness, merely following auditory training curricula is not enough. Phonological and phonemic awareness are metacognitive ("thinking about thinking") skills involving both perceiving sounds in words and manipulating these sounds in important ways. Most of the activities that are involved in phonological and phonemic awareness could and should be incorporated into auditory lessons and learning activities, but most auditory development curricula do not include all the activities involved in phonological and phonemic awareness. Teachers must look through both auditory development and phonemic awareness curricula to incorporate both activities into lessons.

Fluency

Reading fluency is defined as the speed and accuracy (including prosody) with which a child reads, and is based on the assumption that the child is reading known vocabulary and known grammar. One procedure for helping children improve their fluency involves selecting reading materials at their independent reading level and giving them practice reading and rereading. Teachers also provide models of fluent reading and encourage fluency as the students read aloud.

Underlying Assumptions About Fluency

The assumption that repeated reading will improve fluency is a correct assumption only if the developing reader who has a hearing loss understands what she is reading. Fluency cannot be practiced in the absence of comprehension. Consider the teacher who worked with Dauntay. When Dauntay first read the passage, he did not understand the verb idiom "turned on." Because of this, Dauntay did not read the passage with the correct intonation. He paused between the words "turned" and "on" rather than reading the words together. This is because fluency involves phrasing and intonation.

Comprehension is dependent upon knowledge of one's language, including vocabulary and grammar. This is a second assumption that we cannot make with students with hearing loss. Activities to develop fluency and automaticity must be practiced only with material composed of vocabulary and grammar that the child already comprehends. If a passage contains more than one or two words that the child does not know, this passage should not be used to practice fluency.

A third assumption is that the child can group words into phrases when a set of words has been decoded. This does not happen automatically, and children with hearing loss tend to be word callers. Automaticity should be practiced at all levels during the process of learning to read. Address fluency at the beginning levels of sound-symbol association, moving on to syllables, words, and phrases. Practice in quickly reading and rereading smaller units such as phrases will support development of fluency with larger units such as sentences and paragraphs.

The reason we work toward fluency is that readers who are automatically decoding words can use their cognitive energy to comprehend what they are reading. Fluent readers use sound-symbol skills to decode words quickly and hold the essence of the words' meaning in their memory. Fluent readers use phonological skills to manipulate phonemes and shift sounds when misreading a word. For example, if the reader misreads the word "bottle" as "battle" in the sentence: "The general carried the bottle down the hill." If the next sentence were: "He dropped it, and shards of glass flew across the grass," the fluent reader would detect a problem with comprehension. This reader would look back to the word that led to the mistake and make a shift in which phoneme to attach to the vowel.

Vocabulary Comprehension

In the beginning stages when learning to decode words, young children with normal hearing are decoding known words for the most part. They have the prior knowledge of a concept and the prior language to express their world knowledge.

Underlying Assumptions About Vocabulary Comprehension

The first assumption we make about teaching new vocabulary to a child with a hearing loss is that we can teach this vocabulary by relating new words to already mastered concepts. With children who are deaf or hard of hearing, we cannot assume that they understand the old concepts we are using to teach the new. Children with hearing loss have a quantitative deficit in vocabulary (breadth or number of words known) and also a qualitative deficit (depth of understanding of a word). Lack of the words used to teach a new word compounds the vocabulary deficit. Although the child who is deaf or hard of hearing may have seen a knife, fork, spoon, dump truck, and dentist, she may not necessarily have had the opportunity to hear, overhear, and learn by "auditory osmosis" (i.e., incidental learning) what the words for those entities were. Even if she does have someone to share this information with her, she may not have heard a complete message, especially if she was not consistently using hearing technology at a very young age. She may tend to interact with these objects visually rather than auditorily. She may be able to use a fork, but she may not have heard anyone tell her that there is a salad fork, why you shouldn't use a fork if it drops on the floor, or that a farmer uses a pitchfork. This leaves her without the vocabulary necessary to build on or to support typical early childhood education experiences.

A final problem we face with learning vocabulary is that there is not a simple one-to-one correspondence between a word and its meaning. Words can have more than one meaning. Take, for example, the word "run." As a noun, run can refer to a flaw in one's hosiery or something that occurs over an extended period

Figure 5.3   Making a Connection Between an Object and Pictures in the Story

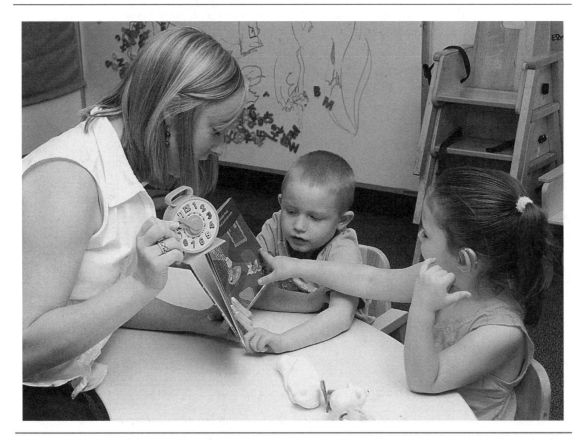

SOURCE: Photographed by John Zimmermann.

of time, as in "the movie had a long run." As a verb, run can refer to the action of running, or it can refer to what your nose does when you have allergies, or it can refer to what a candidate does when he seeks office. "Run" can have a different meaning when paired with different prepositions such as "a run in," referring to an altercation; "a runoff," referring to a second round of voting; or "the run off," referring to the pesticides that wash into lakes and streams. "Run" can also have abstract meanings when placed in such phrases as in "run of the mill" or "run off your mouth." Multiple meanings of words, idiomatic expressions, figures of speech, and nuances of language make reading difficult. If there were a one-to-one correspondence, then learning language and reading would be easy. Since there is no way that we can directly teach a young child every multiple meaning or turn of a phrase or nuance by making him memorize a list of words and word meanings, we must again turn to everyday human interaction for the solution. Conversation about anything and everything all the time is fundamental to the language learning process, and consequently, the language reading process.

Text Comprehension

Text comprehension skills rely on four components: (1) the ability to rapidly decode and attach meaning to known words; (2) the syntactic and morphologic competence to gain collective meaning from the decoded words; (3) the ability to hold the meaning in working memory while processing new words; and (4) the ability to apply text processing strategies for the purpose of figuring out unfamiliar words and passages. Some early reading material has been carefully controlled to account for the developing reader's maturing vocabulary and syntax, but few age-appropriate books are available for the child who has significant delays in the development of grammar.

Underlying Assumptions About Text Comprehension

An assumption often made with normally developing readers is that they have a mature system of grammar (morphology and syntax). Our underlying grammar provides a framework from which we can make assumptions about a word from context (e.g., Hmm . . . I have used my phonics skills to decode this word, *parse*, but I am not sure what it means. Looking at the rest of the sentence, it seems that it could mean cut. Let's go with that. . . .). We cannot make the assumption that children who are deaf and hard of hearing have the underlying grammatical facility needed to fine-tune their best guesses at unknown words. Children may come to the reading process with developing grammar or with no grammar at all if they have not had early intervention. Reading instruction for students who are deaf or hard of hearing must include a carefully planned, sequentially based, intensive intervention to strengthen their weak grammar bases, as described in earlier sections of this book. This intervention must begin as soon as the child is identified as having a hearing loss, whether that is at birth, at age three, or at age 12.

Another assumption made about students learning to read is that teaching them reading strategies will help them understand what they read. Some of these strategies include understanding story structure, making predictions, determining main idea, and generating questions. Reading strategies are based on a metacognitive awareness of the reading process (Schirmer, 2003) and are therefore higher-order thinking skills. One's ability to think is integrally associated with one's language (see Chapter 6). Children who have not had direct instruction to improve their grammar and associated thinking skills may not have the necessary metalinguistic ("thinking about language") skills needed to examine the phrase or sentence they are reading in order to understand and apply reading strategies. In addition, good readers modify their prior impression (inferences) as they go along, based on new information. Struggling readers are so busy attempting to apply the strategies they have learned that they don't modify their perceptions based on new inferences.

Reading is an interactive process. Effective readers think while manipulating text (Scharer, Pinnell, Lyons, & Fountas, 2005). This requires a large memory that can store the ideas expressed by the printed message while scanning through a mental list of choices of possible interpretations and considering possible meanings that would result (see Figure 5.4).

Figure 5.4   Process Involved in Applying Interpretations

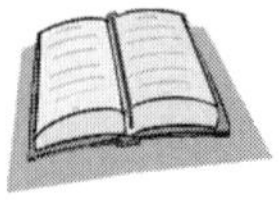	**Step 1:** The child reads words (relying on rapid word recognition skills and fluency) and holds them in memory.
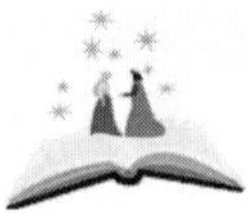 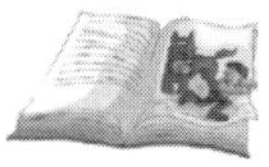	**Step 2:** Considers possible interpretations.
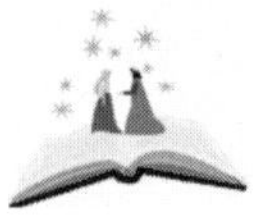	**Step 3:** Chooses the meaning based on the possible interpretations, and applies it.
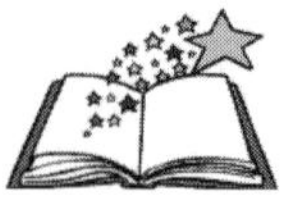	**Step 4:** Thinks up a new meaning based on prior knowledge and text review if the text still makes no sense.

This is a very time-costly and mental resource-costly process for any reader. It assumes that the child has the prior world knowledge, the vocabulary, the grammar, the memory, and the metacognitive and metalinguistic skills necessary to keep cycling through the process until meaning has been extracted. This is even more of a challenge for developing readers with hearing losses. Teachers who are working with developing readers must ensure that comprehension is accessible at the end of the reading lesson. Any strategies that are taught must be set in the context of the student's linguistic capacity. A teacher must also ensure that the strategy being taught (e.g., predicting) has been practiced verbally, before applying it to the reading task. The teacher must then structure the lessons so that the strategy proves effective in helping the students understand what they are reading.

Additional Assumptions

We must also consider some additional assumptions about the language and literacy learning process in general in order to understand the challenges facing children with hearing losses as they learn to read. These issues are more deafness related than literacy related.

One assumption made about struggling readers is that they need to catch up to the skills of good readers and that this can be done by intensively talking to them. The issue for the typical struggling reader is one of *catching up* to what others know. The issue for children who are deaf or hard of hearing is more one of *catching on* than catching up. The available auditory signals are not complete messages. They have to work harder to catch on to what is being said and read.

We need to talk a lot to the deaf and hard of hearing child, but that is not enough. We must also present language systematically. Stimulating language development with a child who is deaf or hard of hearing is not just talking more; it involves analyzing the child's language understanding and use and providing opportunities for communicating with the language structures and vocabulary the child needs to develop.

Children with hearing loss need intensive spoken language stimulation at the sound level presented to them in a very systematic and analytical way. This is different from how children with normal hearing learn to deal with the sounds of their language. Children with normal hearing learn words holistically and then analyze them for reading purposes. When children with hearing loss receive intensive auditory stimulation, they may learn the sounds in words before beginning the reading process. They can then put them together for language learning purposes. Sounds are highly organized for the child who is getting a precise, orderly exposure to speech. Children with hearing losses who have had significant auditory stimulation bring great skills to the task of decoding. These advanced auditory skills result in an ability to perceive new words that is different from those of struggling readers with normal hearing. The struggling reader with normal hearing may hear a word as a whole but have trouble perceiving the sounds in a word; the child with a hearing loss understands sounds in words, but may be functioning with an incomplete message. If he has had a systematic exposure to speech sounds, he may think more analytically than holistically. On the other hand, many children with hearing losses do not have this intensive auditory intervention. If these students have not had a systematic exposure to speech sounds, then they have an ineffective and inefficient system for listening to new words. Instructors must determine if it would be more appropriate to teach these students to read through visual means.

Another assumption pertains to the use of habilitation versus rehabilitation approaches. The assumption is that the struggling student needs more information than just auditory information to analyze the words of his language. The important issue here is that there is a difference between *habilitation* and *remedial* approaches. Habilitation is a concept that is unfamiliar to most general education teachers, but for teachers who work with students with hearing loss, this is essential. We are not teaching the same things to a child who is deaf or hard of hearing as we are to a struggling reader who can hear. When language or concepts or auditory skills do not exist, we need to focus specifically on what is lacking and build that up. This is habilitation. In multi-sensory remedial programs, the normally hearing child receives more and more cues and clues that will help him access his known language. By adding more cues and clues for the child who is deaf or hard of hearing, we may be only increasing the burden of unknown information he must figure out. For example, some remedial programs add labels for sounds, key words, or other language-rich mnemonics. However, if the child is deaf and does not have the vocabulary or general knowledge background to understand the label, key word, or mnemonic, then this approach may be counterproductive. Programs that depend on mnemonics may rely on too much verbal mediation that takes up extra cognitive energy. There are cases when parts of multisensory programs are helpful, especially when the child may have a specific reading disability in addition to a hearing loss, but we need to evaluate each child carefully to determine which parts to use and not use.

An additional assumption that teachers need to modify is the proper use of published lists of common words to develop word reading. Teachers who have deaf or hard of hearing students in their classrooms need to get their first hundred reading words from a *spoken* vocabulary list so that they will be learning to read words that they can most easily comprehend. The MacArthur-Bates Communicative Development Inventories (CDI Advisory Committee, 2003) provide lists of spoken vocabulary that develop in children with normal hearing. Word lists, such as the Dolch list (Dolch, 1948), consist of many common words, but Dolch words are also very heavy on connecting concepts (e.g., of, and, will). These kinds of words are devoid of meaning in and of themselves and, for a child with a hearing loss, may not yet be a part of the child's oral language. Decoding of these words is best learned first in the context of a phrase or sentence, surrounded by words that convey a more concrete meaning. Teaching a child to read words in his spoken vocabulary, alongside a phonics program such as the "Children's Early Intervention for Speech-Language-Reading" program (Tade & Vitali, 1994) helps develop sight words and phonics skills, both of which are necessary for children who are deaf and hard of hearing.

USING READING TO DEVELOP LANGUAGE—A PARADOX

At the beginning of this chapter we stressed that a child must be able to comprehend what he is reading. We said that the beginning reader must be presented only with text that is within the child's vocabulary and language level. But after the student has developed an understanding of the reading process and facility with reading tasks, the opposite is also true. Teachers who work with children with hearing losses often use reading as a tool to teach the children the details of their language. We can use the printed version of words with deaf and hard of hearing children to teach unknown words. At the same time that we are working on meaning, we can use print to teach the pronunciation of the words. As long as we control for vocabulary and sentence structure when we are developing reading, we do not wait until the elementary-age child with a hearing loss has mastered age-appropriate vocabulary and grammar to start the reading process. Once the student understands the reading task, reading becomes a tool for learning language. For example, the -ing ending on a word may be difficult to access through hearing, and is difficult to see on the lips, so the first time many deaf and hard of hearing children get access to it is when they see it in print. It is not uncommon for children who are deaf and hard of hearing to learn -ing by reading it. Reading can be used to develop language.

Reading also serves as an important tool for developing vocabulary for children who are deaf and hard of hearing. Students with normal hearing acquire most of their vocabulary by hearing it spontaneously from others until third grade, at which time print teaches them new vocabulary. Prior to this time they are called to read vocabulary they already know. Around third grade, they are reading new vocabulary and learning it through the printed word. Students who are deaf or hard of hearing also learn vocabulary and language through their reading. Teachers of the deaf and hard of hearing use reading as an invaluable tool to give students access to things they don't hear. Reading *becomes* a visual tool that is of great importance to a teacher of the deaf especially in helping children who are deaf or hard of hearing move past the telegraphic stage in their language development.

We would like to make one final point about children with hearing losses who come late to the reading process. These children require intensive language-based instruction to develop a language foundation upon which to build their reading skills. Each child acquires information through his personal filters, which are a function of how his brain is organized. Older students who are deaf (and communicating through a visual system—sign language or home signs) filter information through a brain that has not been organized around listening or a spoken language function. Their brains think in terms of visual organization and in the matching of new visual patterns to old visual patterns. They therefore have a different organization of language than people who have organized language through listening. Consider whether a student who is deaf is an auditory learner or a visual learner when determining the most effective approach to teaching. A six-year-old who is deaf and has never been exposed to any spoken language is most likely going to depend on the strengths of her visual frameworks and filters. A four-year-old who was born deaf and is a new listener because he has just received a cochlear implant will benefit from highly structured auditory input. We should tap into what he already has in his visual systems and build a bridge between the auditory and the visual systems.

ASSESSMENT

Our purpose in this section is not to present an exhaustive list of all reading assessment tools available but to highlight the two keys to a good literacy assessment with children who are deaf and hard of hearing: (1) pair literacy assessment with a good language assessment, and (2) focus on progress relative to self rather than relative to others.

Since the underlying language system of children with hearing loss can be missing so many elements, it is essential to know what skills a child has in both his spoken language repertoire and his reading repertoire. For example, let's look at Maggie's assessment results for vocabulary. (See assessment results in Table 5.3.) These scores tell us that there is a mismatch between Maggie's present spoken vocabulary and the vocabulary she needs in order to be able to discuss even the simplest book used in the classroom. Collaboration among the parents, teacher, and speech-language pathologist is needed to chart a course for improving Maggie's basic vocabulary and language skills, and reading instruction must be modified to be presented within Maggie's listening and language ability as discussed earlier in the chapter.

Table 5.3   Summary of Maggie's Test Results

Category	Results
Placement	Kindergarten
Johns Basic Reading Inventory	Independent Reading Level: Unscorable
	Instructional Reading Level: Pre-preprimer
MacArthur-Bates Communicative Development Inventory: Words and Sentences	Age Score: 24 months

In addition to the formal data available from the tests given in Table 5.3, we need to find out how Maggie interacts with printed materials themselves. What kind of print matter draws Maggie's attention? Does she seem to benefit from looking at pictures and other contextual cues? Does she have any systematic approach to attacking a word she does not know, or are her efforts random rather than trial-and-error? Does she ask for help appropriately if she does not know a word, or does she give up easily? There are several good checklists that we can use to discern information pertaining to a young child's motivation to read and motivation to figure out the missing pieces (Metsala, McCann, & Dacey, 1997). In addition, a teacher can use story retelling to get an important estimate of how much information a student retains from a reading passage (Strong, 1998).

No matter what the age of the child, be sure to request a comprehensive language assessment to pair with your reading assessments. Keep the child's present vocabulary and grammar levels foremost in your mind as you review materials and make decisions about which to choose and how to present new literacy skills.

IMPLICATIONS FOR THE SPECIAL EDUCATION TEACHER

Almost all children who are deaf or hard of hearing will need assistance in learning to read. Systematic and analytic approaches to listening are very important for children who are deaf or hard of hearing to develop an auditory base for spoken language. Children acquire listening and language skills in a developmental sequence. That sequence has to be enhanced for the child who is deaf or hard of hearing. This systematic development must start at the beginning level, no matter what age a child is. If a student is four years old and has not yet mastered listening skills associated with two-year-olds, then intervention needs to begin at the two-year-old level and provide intensive stimulation to move him forward through the normal developmental sequence. The sequence we follow is typical, but the approach we use is not. Most children who are deaf or hard of hearing hear the teacher's instructions in a degraded signal. The teacher's job is to find ways to help increase and refine the children's range of perception, to bridge the gap while they are learning listening and speaking strategies, and to assist the general education teacher in making necessary accommodations.

Teachers providing support services need to think systematically about the kind of instruction a child has received in the past. If the child has not had carefully planned instruction in listening to the sounds of speech, begin here. If the child has had a lot of listening training but still is not connecting to print, then use a curriculum such as the "Children's Early Intervention for Speech-Language-Reading" program (Tade & Vitali, 1994). It is often the correct choice to begin phonics instruction with the long vowels (and diphthongs) instead of consonants because these phonemes are more audible. When selecting consonants to introduce, the teacher may first choose to teach those consonants that are more audible and distinguishable from each other auditorily, such as /m/ versus /sh/. See Chapter 6 for information on the audibility of the speech sounds.

Everyone involved in a child's educational program needs to make sure that the child is mastering an ever-increasing vocabulary base. This requires the careful effort of those who have a clear understanding of the vocabulary that the child has mastered. This effort can be successful only through extensive record keeping. Additional work on vocabulary expansion (i.e., multiple meanings, idiomatic and figurative uses, abstract connotations) must continue throughout the school years for a student with a hearing loss because there are many levels of knowledge of a word. He might have a specific meaning for the word, but may not know the nuances of the word.

Instruction in new vocabulary must begin with teaching the concepts behind the words and then all the age-appropriate variations of meaning. One person must accept the responsibility of determining the vocabulary, grammar, and underlying concepts that the child has missed, then planning and organizing the development of these skills and concepts, carefully coordinating the efforts of all involved in the child's education (teachers, therapists, family members). This solid foundation will support the child as she learns to read.

IMPLICATIONS FOR THE GENERAL EDUCATION TEACHER

The general education teacher needs to work closely with the teacher of the deaf and speech-language pathologist. The general education teacher needs to gain an understanding of the child's current level of vocabulary and language. Screen any decoding activities, reading material, and work pages that are used in the classroom so that the words given to the student to decode are meaningful. The general education teacher must work closely with the teacher of the deaf and speech-language pathologist to understand the compensatory strategies that should be incorporated into communication with the child who is deaf or hard of hearing to help bridge the gap between what is being said and what the child is hearing.

INTERVENTION

The remainder of this chapter presents techniques and strategies for intervention at the different developmental stages.

Infants and Toddlers

The following list identifies language activities that parents can do at home with their infants and toddlers to encourage communication development and to lay down the foundation for the listening and language base necessary to develop reading.

1. Talk without ceasing to infants and toddlers. Talk about what you are doing when you are doing it. Talk in short phrases using lots of intonation and emotion. As the baby or toddler gets older, use longer and longer sentences. This will give him the language base needed for later reading.

2. Use books as a way to talk with infants and toddlers. Every bookstore and discount chain has a section of baby books. Any book with nice pictures and clear action will do. Little babies will use their books for teething rings, but that's OK. They will also look at the pictures. Talk about the pictures, then talk about them some more.

3. Point out words in the infant's or toddler's environment. Show her your name on the mailbox. Show her the name of her favorite cereal every time you pour a bowl. Show her the name brand on her sneakers every time you pick them up.

4. As your toddler starts to pretend to read, point out different words in books that are related directly to pictures in the books.

Preschoolers

In addition to the activities above, add the following activities for preschool-age children. Our purpose in these suggestions is for you to be able to expand the child's spoken language. This is not intended as a comprehensive curriculum. If you are looking for a curriculum guide for preschool children with hearing loss, consider some of the suggestions mentioned in the Resources section of this book. The ideas in the next two sections are not new. We have gleaned them from years of experience as well as the works of others (e.g., Fountas & Pinnell, 1996; McAnally, Rose, & Quigley, 1999; Schirmer, 2000; Schleper, 1997; clerccenter.gallaudet.edu/Literacy/index.html).

Read, read, and read to your children who are deaf and hard of hearing. This is a great way to expose them to concepts, vocabulary, and grammar. Anderson, Wilson, and Fielding (1988) demonstrated that the more minutes a child spends in reading each day, the higher their percentile scores on standardized tests. We must not underestimate the value of exposure to text.

1. Read stories daily. Discuss the concepts. Act them out using props.

2. Point to words as you are reading them.

3. Make sure that you are reading not only things that they know about and care about but also things that will expand their experiences.

4. Help students visualize what they are reading. Create mental images.

5. Read a variety of materials, including but not limited to stories and information. Consider all the things that people read: newspapers, cereal boxes and food packages, captions, road signs, menus, pagers, personal data devices, lists describing items down store aisles, e-mail, instant messages, medicine bottles, junk mail, magazines, cookbooks and other how-to books and manuals, wordless picture books and games.

6. Read for a variety of purposes, including: information/instructional, enjoyment, survival/daily living, technology/communications. Spend time on modeling real-world reading for the child.

7. Mediate what you are reading to the child through your personal experiences. Talk about what you thought and felt. It does not matter how you expand on the ideas, just as long as you expand on them. Connect what you say to the child's life.

8. Include the parents and siblings as reading partners. Show parents how to read to their children. Invite parents to come in and read to the preschool class.

9. Expand vocabulary beyond what you are teaching to associated concepts. For example, if you are working on "apple," expose the child also to "peel," "seed," and "core."

10. Teach supraordinate categories. A child may know "apple," "banana," and "orange," but she might not know "fruit."

11. Make the implied obvious. Use scaffolding (unknown-known-unknown sequence) to make this connection. Say the sentence as written, then say the implied information, followed by the sentence as written as in, "Two more went to the kitchen with her. Two more bunnies went to the kitchen. Two more went to the kitchen with her."

12. Help them make connections from what they are reading to their real world. Follow the child's lead as she discusses tangential thoughts, and keep connecting her back to the story and to the words on the page.

13. Reread the same books over and over to young children. Kids want to hear the same story over and over again. As you work on the different

intricacies of reading, they are working from a known base and are expanding their skills (known-unknown-known sequence).

14. Keep materials available so children can reread by themselves and read to each other.

15. Read books with rhyming or repetitive patterns. After the child is familiar with the book, pause before saying the rhyming word or repeating phrase and see if the child can fill in the rhyming or repeating word. Dr. Seuss is great for this.

16. Adjust your body position, facial expression, and tone of voice to represent the story. Represent all the emotions and make all characterizations clear.

17. Expose the child to concepts of print such as: cover, title, author, illustrator, beginning, ending, left/right orientation, top/bottom orientation, letters differ from words, letters have order, there are capitals and lower case letters, empty spaces mark beginning and end of words, printed words relate to spoken words, capitals at beginning, and punctuation.

18. Model literate behaviors. Reading should be a social conversation event. Expand the preschooler's social world through reading in small groups.

19. Explain the purpose of the text. This can be done very naturally and simply. Read a variety of materials and explain why you are reading them. For example, "I'm reading the directions on the soup can label. The label tells me how to cook the soup." Or, "I'm reading a letter from the principal. The letter says that picture day is next week."

20. Write things down for the purpose of reading them later (e.g., the daily schedule of class activities). Make a scrapbook and write labels for the pictures. Write a note for the child to take to another person. For example, a teacher can say, "I'm writing a note to Mr. Smith that says, 'Dear Mr. Smith, May I borrow your stapler? Your friend, Mrs. Jones.' Please give Mr. Smith the note."

21. Turn on the captions on your television. Many programs and movies are captioned. Even before children can decode the words, they become familiar with the concept that the print they see on the TV screen is related to the words they are hearing.

Children in the Primary Grades

By now you will be starting to use traditional materials that are available for all kindergarten and first-grade children. Work closely with your consultants to make sure that the child in your class has the necessary prerequisite language and hearing skills to do the tasks associated with these materials.

1. Ask for an evaluation of the deaf or hard of hearing child's present vocabulary skills. If your student does not have age-appropriate vocabulary, make sure that an IEP meeting happens so that appropriate,

intensive language instruction can begin. This should involve specialized help outside of your classroom as well as collaboration to assist you in knowing how best to communicate with the child in your classroom.

2. Ask for an evaluation of the child's present grammar skills. The Preschool Language Scale (see Resource B) is a good test to use to screen whether the child has key grammatical structures associated with the simple sentence stage. If your student does not have most of the grammar associated with the simple sentence level (see Table 2.4), then ask for an IEP review to consider the need for special services from a teacher of the deaf and speech-language pathologist.

3. Ask for a comprehensive evaluation of the child's present listening skills. Depending on the child's aided responses to sound, you may want to consider an alternative sequence of working on phonemic awareness to the sequence presented in traditional materials. Review the information in Chapters 1 and 6 on the formant frequencies associated with speech sounds. If the student you are working with does not have high-frequency hearing, he may have difficulty in hearing the difference between the sounds you are working on for phonemic awareness. For example, it is easier to discriminate (hear the difference between) the words "black" and "blue" than it is to hear the difference between the words "red" and "green" because there is a larger difference in the first formants between -a- and -oo- than there is between -e- and -ee-. Work with your consultants to make sure that you are presenting tasks to the child in a sequence that he can easily follow based on the amount of his residual hearing.

4. When planning the stories that you will read to the class or use in your lessons, be sure to give a copy to the speech-language pathologist and teacher of the deaf to look through the books and identify the vocabulary and grammar that will be a challenge to the child. The teacher or speech-language pathologist may decide to work with your student beforehand to teach vocabulary and concepts or may give you suggestions for teaching these.

5. Recognize that language, thinking, and literacy go hand in hand. Use literacy activities to encourage the child to think. Talk about higher-order concepts represented in the book such as time, space, description, sequence, problem solving, cause-effect relationships, procedural thinking, categorization, inference and implication, and abstractions.

6. Use journals as ways to increase the child's vocabulary. Increase vocabulary and model correct language structures by writing reflective sentences and comments on the content of the child's journal.

7. When reading stories to the student, provide grammar bridges. Use simpler grammar to bridge to difficult grammar. Break the story into smaller sentences. Notice in the following example that by eliminating the slashed words and adding in some others [ ], you can use natural breaks and produce simpler sentences than the long one in the actual story. Removable tape can be applied to hide words you have chosen to discard.

Poor little Cottontail was very tired, ~~for~~ this was the first time she had ever gone so far or so fast in her life, ~~and~~ she was beginning to hope that she could soon take the little basket ~~that~~ [The basket] was set aside for her own children ~~and~~ [She wanted to] go hopping home, ~~when~~ [Then] old, wise, kind Grandfather called her to him.

After the child reads and comprehends the simpler grammar, give the child the opportunity to read the original version.

8. Address potential word meaning breakdowns before they happen. Anticipate upcoming problems (e.g., "Oh, there is a very funny word on the next page. It is 'anemone.' You are going to read the word 'anemone.'").

9. Call attention to whole word strategy errors (e.g., says "smell" for "shell"). Praise the child's efforts (You're right! It does look like "smell."). Write *m* and *h* and reinforce her for seeing the similarities, then explain the difference and have her say the word correctly. Draw the child's attention to the letters within the word.

10. Call the child's attention to semantic substitutions strategy errors (e.g., says "hot" for "burn"). Praise his effort. ("Yes, you know they are talking about a fire. That's right. A fire is very hot. But what happens if you touch a fire? What do you get? You get a burn. B-U-R-N. Show me the word 'burn.'")

11. Delay teaching the child the names of the letters of the alphabet. It is more important for him to learn the sounds. In order to proceed with phonemic awareness and phonics, he must know the sound of the letters. Once he has mastered the sounds, he may more easily be able to learn that each letter has a name.

12. As with your work on activities requiring perception of differences among speech sounds, ensure that the consonant sound differences you are working on are within the child's listening range. Refer to the strong and weak consonant charts in Chapter 1.

13. When learning a sound, show kids all the orthographic versions simultaneously. Tell them, for example, "It sounds like -ee- but here are other ways you can spell it." Don't expect students to learn all the spellings at once, but begin to expose examples systematically to them as they occur in the books you are using. Keep a chart of all the different spellings you have covered. Maintain a log that travels with the student from one year to the next. Have the students develop their own pronunciation dictionaries containing words in alphabetical order that have the same sound as the main vowel on the dictionary page as you see in Figure 5.5.

Figure 5.5   William's Vocabulary Log

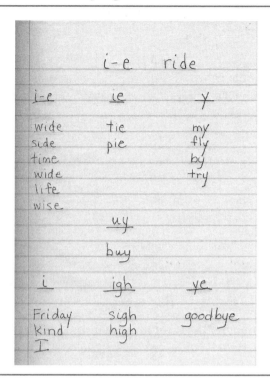

SOURCE: Used with permission.

14. Build a lexicon of sight words at the automatic word recognition level in conjunction with working on phonics, and develop the words that will be used in phonics instruction activities into the child's known, automatic lexicon. This means that your first months of reading instruction may focus on vocabulary rather than phonemic awareness or phonics, but your phonics instruction will be more meaningful if you are working on words that the child knows and understands.

15. Good phonics instruction does not overly rely on memorization of rules. Commonly taught rules rarely apply to more than 75 percent of the words. For example, "When two vowels go walking, the first one does the talking" is true only 50 percent of the time.

16. Understand that there are many curriculum guides that you can adapt for children who are deaf or hard of hearing but that none will meet the needs of all children. Keep a collection of other products handy (see Resources section).

17. Starting from a base of known vocabulary and known grammar (or the child's independent reading level), work directly on the development of fluency skills at all levels (sounds, syllables, words, phrases, sentences,

paragraphs) through such techniques as independent practice and rereading, auditory modeling, reader's theater, repeated readings, and phrase-cued texts.

18. Include the use of captioned materials (www.cfv.org) in content area lessons. Parents report that their deaf children learn words from captions very quickly. Children see the caption and use the context to help them figure out the word, which promotes comprehension of what they are seeing on TV.

19. Teach reading strategies that are appropriate for the age and skill level of the student such as using prior knowledge, predicting, identifying the main idea and summarization, questioning, clarifying, making inferences, and visualizing.

20. Take care when using story maps and story grammar to help students visualize different themes and genres of writing. Focus on one theme and read multiple books on that same theme, discussing the elements of the story map and story grammar.

21. Start early to build the awareness that the structure of expository text (i.e., textbooks) is different from the structure of literary text. Expository text has as its purpose the explanation of facts and concepts. It informs, persuades, and explains. Common text structures include but are not limited to: compare/contrast, cause-effect, description, and time order. Expository text also provides additional information through the use of headings, subheadings, signal words (words in bold or italics), and picture captions. Some begin with objective statements and some end with questions for review. You will not get to this level of reading instruction until the end of the elementary years, but it is never too soon to start exposing the child to these in routine, everyday reading activities. The use of instruction manuals is particularly helpful.

THE LITERACY TEAM

A key to the development of reading in a child who has a hearing loss is to consider the process a team effort and a multiyear effort. Continually attaching spoken language development to literacy in the real world must be the responsibility of everyone involved. Parents must understand the teacher's reading objectives so they can use real-world reading such as food labels, menus, and magazines in the home to reinforce these. Teachers must understand the experiences the child has at home in order to incorporate these into language and reading lessons in the classroom. Speech-language pathologists must understand the language demands of the classroom so they can prepare the child to handle these. When a child comes from a non-English-speaking family, collaboration with a specialist in cultural expectations of the family is essential in maintaining positive home-school relationships. Opening and maintaining the lines of communication between home and school should be a primary objective for all team members.

In addition to viewing literacy as a multidisciplinary team effort, one must also view services to a child with a hearing loss from a multiyear perspective. Depending on how late the child came to the language-learning process, the child's acquisition of speech, language, and literacy skills is going to require a much closer scrutiny that those of a child with normal hearing. Clear records need to be maintained, and these records need to go from teacher to teacher and from year to year.

SUMMARY

This chapter described the process of learning to read, the factors that lead to success in reading, and the effect that a hearing loss can have on an individual's ability to learn to read. An overarching difference between the processes by which children with and without hearing learn to read is the interdependency of spoken language and literacy in reading development. Young children who are deaf or hard of hearing are often learning to read while simultaneously learning to communicate.

The factors that lead to reading success for typically developing children are also factors that lead to success for children with hearing loss; however, we must look at these factors from a different perspective. Certainly phonological awareness, vocabulary development, comprehension strategies, and fluency skills must be taught, but they must be taught with careful consideration given to each individual child's present levels of performance on listening, speaking, and language. This chapter examined the assumptions that underlie the above-mentioned skills and provided guidance regarding how they must be approached given the influences of a hearing loss. In addition, we discussed issues surrounding assessment and the need to view literacy development in children with hearing loss from a multiyear, team perspective. Finally, we presented strategies that teachers of children from infancy through later elementary school age may employ to ensure continued literacy growth.

Children who are deaf and hard of hearing are often learning language at the same time as they are learning to read. In many instances, reading becomes one of the tools by which they learn language. Therefore, there is a unique, reciprocal relationship between language and reading for children with hearing loss that is unlike the relationship that the child with normal hearing experiences. Teachers must keep this language/reading interrelationship clearly in the forefront of all that they are doing to ensure that the young child with a hearing loss is making daily progress in both language and reading skill development.

Part 2

The Science of Intervention

Now that you have reviewed the "*what*" and the "*how*" of intervention and have artfully applied many of the practices and strategies, you will want to take a look at the science underlying the art. This explains the "*why*" of intervention. The better you understand the science behind recommended techniques and strategies, the better you will be able to apply those techniques and strategies.

Part 2 is composed of one relatively long chapter. This chapter, *How Children Hear and Talk: Fundamentals of Listening and Speaking,* explains the science behind speech, hearing, listening devices, and classroom acoustics.

How Children Hear and Talk **6**

Fundamentals of Listening and Speaking

In this chapter you will learn about how we listen and speak, the anatomy of hearing, the linguistics of spoken language, how hearing is measured, the listening devices that are available to assist children, how to set up environments that support listening, and how to monitor listening performance.

THE SPEECH CHAIN

In order to develop spoken language, children must coordinate a very complex set of systems. *The Speech Chain* (Denes & Pinson, 1993; see Figure 6.1) is a good tool to help you picture the different parts of spoken communication and how they work together as a smooth, integrated process. First, we have a thought. We think about something: ice cream, a massage, the grocery list. These thoughts are organized at the *Linguistic Level* and then put into the code of language (i.e., words and grammar). Next, the brain takes this coded thought (e.g., "Hmmm. Ice cream would taste good right about now!") and develops a set of instructions for the lungs, larynx, tongue, and so forth on how to produce the words, "Hmmm. Ice cream would taste good right about now!" The brain sends commands to the lungs, voice, tongue, and so forth through neural impulses. These nerve impulses cause appropriate movement of the muscles of speech. The nerve impulses and muscle movements are *Physiological Level* actions. The flow of breath and vocal vibration made at the physiological level cause changes in air pressure, creating a sound wave. We call this the *Acoustic Level* because sound waves travel through the air from the mouth of the speaker to the ears of the listener. Once the sound wave reaches the listener, we say it is at the *Physiological Level* again because the sound wave (which is actually a change in air pressure) activates a chain reaction of mechanisms in the ear that interact with the auditory nerve (i.e., the main nerve for hearing). By now the wave has been transformed from a wave of sound pressure to nerve impulses, which travel up the auditory nerve to the brain, bringing us back to the *Linguistic Level.* Once the stimulus is back at this level, our brain perceives these nerve impulses as sounds. At this level the brain interprets sounds as word sequences (Hmmm. Ice cream would taste good right about now!), using the listener's knowledge of the communication system (Oh. She wants some ice cream!), and the rules of language (Oh. We're talking about ice cream, not about fishing tackle!), to help the brain understand and respond to the speaker's message.

Figure 6.1   The Speech Chain

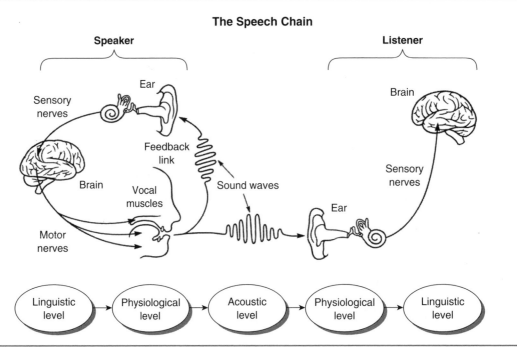

SOURCE: From *The Speech Chain: The Physics and Biology of Spoken Language* by Peter B. Denes and Elliott N. Pinson, copyright © 1993 by W. H. Freeman and Company. Reprinted by permission of Henry Holt and Company, LLC.

In the remainder of this chapter we present a deeper discussion of each of the levels and emphasize *essential practices* associated with each level. Communication has both receptive (listening and understanding) and expressive (producing) components. The speech chain presents aspects of expressive language on the left and receptive language on the right. We discuss aspects of the speech chain from the outside of the figure in toward the middle; that is, we discuss both receptive and expressive linguistic skills in one section, receptive and expressive aspects of physiology in another section, and aspects of acoustics including listening devices and classroom acoustics in another section.

LINGUISTIC LEVEL

In order to provide instruction in spoken language, it is important for the teacher to understand the components of the linguistic level.

The linguistics behind spoken language allows us to be creative language users. One's knowledge of the rules of language is not based on having heard a sentence before. Consider the sentence: *Twelve old alligators with no teeth swam under my yacht.* Although you have never heard this sentence before, it makes complete sense. Knowledge of a language makes it possible to understand and produce new sentences. Human language gives us the ability to communicate about our experiences, to converse about past and future, to convey information about things that are far away and even to share things that exist only in our imagination. The grammar associated with language use is often called *generative grammar,* which is a set of rules that allow us to "generate" new sentences. Language is considered to be made up of five major systems.

Essential Practice #1

> Language is made up of five major systems. A breakdown in any of the systems will influence all the other systems. Children must learn the rules of each system.

Language is like a complicated card game. This game has rules that all the players know. The rules of the game include how the symbols are arranged on each card (morphology), what each card means (semantics), how to combine the cards together to score points (syntax), and the rules for playing the game (pragmatics). (See Table 6.1 for definitions.) If a player doesn't know the rules, the game is over before it starts. If a player breaks one of the rules, the other players will notice. We learn this game by watching others play it and by joining in ourselves. Learning to play the language game develops in stages. These stages are controlled by the child's development: developing a need to communicate, developing the thinking skills to discern the rules, and developing the physical ability to speak clearly. All children follow the same stages of language development in almost exactly the same way no matter what language they are learning.

When we communicate, we knit together these five aspects of language to create meaning. A breakdown or lack in any area of language can affect the communicator's ability both to get his ideas across to others and to understand the meaning of what other people are saying. Children who are deaf or hard of

Table 6.1   Definitions of Language Systems

System	Definition
Semantics	The rules that specify the meanings of words and word combinations
Morphology	The rules of word formation that build words out of pieces
Syntax	The rules governing the combination of words into phrases and sentences
Pragmatics	The social rules for language use
Phonology	The rules for the sound patterns of spoken language

hearing need careful exposure and systematic stimulation to develop expertise in all areas of language.

Essential Practice #2

> The semantic system describes meaning at the word, phrase, and sentence level. Words, phrases, and sentences can have more than one meaning, and meanings can be concrete or abstract.

Knowledge of a language means knowing that certain words signify certain concepts or meanings. The relationship between a word and its *referent* (i.e., the thing to which a word refers) is completely arbitrary. Neither the shape nor physical attributes of an object determines the pronunciation of the word. Semantic knowledge is the understanding of the meaning of words themselves. This includes understanding of the undertones, associations, and unspoken subtext that may be associated with a word or word combination. Semantic knowledge also governs how words can be combined in a meaningful way. For example, consider the following sentence: *My brother is an only child.* All the pieces go together fine; however, because of the meanings of the words, this sentence does not follow the semantic rules for word combination. Because I'm talking about "My brother," he cannot be an "only child." Since semantics is based on the interplay of word meanings, it is a difficult puzzle to unravel for an individual who has a diminished knowledge of word meanings, including multiple meanings for the same word and subtle differences in nuance between words. For example, a deaf adolescent tested the frozen pond before putting on his skates and said, "The ice is powerful. It's okay to skate." His use of the word "powerful" was understandable here, because he had been taught that "powerful" meant "strong." Powerful and strong can be thought of as meaning the same thing, but in this instance, "strong" is the correct word and "powerful" is not.

Semantic understanding also involves being able to derive meaning that is not directly associated with the words used, including multiple meanings of words, idioms, and other figures of speech. A teacher must be very careful when working with a child with a hearing loss to ensure that the child understands the nuances being conveyed by the words being used. A student with a hearing loss may need explicit instruction in all aspects of semantic understanding.

Essential Practice #3

> The morphology system is composed of root words, prefixes, suffixes, and other parts of speech that change the meaning of words. Children must begin to learn about these rules at a very early age.

Understanding the meanings of words requires understanding how small pieces added to or taken away from a word can change the meaning or the part of speech of a word. The creation of words from smaller pieces is studied under the heading of morphology. *Morphemes* are the smallest meaningful pieces into which words can be broken. For example, the word, *runners* has three morphemes. A free morpheme is a part of a word that can be a word all by itself, such as "run." Compound words are made of two free morphemes (e.g., homerun). The other kind of morpheme is a *bound morpheme*, a part of the word that can't stand alone. In our example, *"runners,"* the bound morphemes are: *-er*, and *-s*. Children learning language need to be taught about word roots (e.g., bio- refers to plants and animals), and grammatical (also called *inflectional*) markers representing such concepts as tense, number, gender, person, and infinitive (e.g., I want *to* play.), and derivational prefixes and suffixes (e.g., dis-, un-, -er, -ly). When a child speaks in two- and three-word utterances, he tends to leave off the inflectional morphemes (e.g., Where Daddy go?). We say that this child is using *preinflected grammar.* Understanding of parts of words assists in comprehension of word meanings.

Essential Practice #4

> Syntax refers to the order of words in sentences. Children must hear word order in structured presentations in order to assimilate order into their growing language.

Syntax is the way words are combined and put in order. Syntax affects whether or not a sentence sounds "right" to our ears. Different syntactical combinations can also change the meaning of a sentence. For example, examine the two sentences: *The children sang songs for the teacher. The teacher sang songs for the children.* These two sentences have completely different meanings even though they have exactly the same words. Let's look at the sentence: *Songs sang for the children teacher.* This is the same group of words, but the sentence has no linguistic meaning even though it's made up of meaningful units. Rules of syntax determine how words can combine to express a specific meaning. Competent speakers of a language automatically know what is syntactically correct and what isn't based on an intuitive knowledge of specific rules.

Essential Practice #5

> The pragmatic system is another system of language. This system tells us who can say what to whom, when, where, and how. If a child violates these rules, he is often thought of as "odd" or "rude." Pragmatic skills require direct instruction in most instances.

Pragmatics involves social aspects of language such as how sentences are made to fit in with the flow of a conversation. Examples of pragmatic rule categories are: verbal turn taking, giving appropriate responses, conveying empathy, topic switching, and overture into conversation. Children with hearing losses often benefit from direct instruction in the social aspect of language including keeping on topic, when and how to interject into a conversation, and appropriate language to use in formal and informal situations.

Essential Practice #6

> The phonology system allows us to describe actual speech as separate from language. Children who are deaf or hard of hearing need incidental and didactic instruction in learning the rules of speech.

The basic unit of speech is called the *phoneme*. A phoneme is an individual speech sound such as /b/ as in "buy," /sh/ as in "shoe," or -oo- as in "boo." Phonemes come in two types: (1) vowels and diphthongs, and (2) consonants. There are 42 to 44 speech sounds, depending on local dialect. Vowels and diphthongs are produced by voicing at the vocal cords. Diphthongs are made of two vowels: we start with one vowel (e.g., -o- as in *hot)* and move through a continuous transition to end up as another vowel (e.g., -oo- as in shoe) to make up a diphthong (e.g., in this case, -ou- as in *mouth)*. Consonants are described by the characteristics of manner (i.e., how the air moves through the vocal mechanism), place (i.e., where the articulators of speech are placed), and voicing (i.e., whether the vocal folds vibrate or not). The rules of phonetics govern how phonemes may be combined in different languages to form natural-sounding words, how phonemes are adjusted depending on the speech sounds surrounding them (called *coarticulation*), and patterns of vocal intonation, timing, and stress (called *prosody*). If you have trouble hearing any of the sounds of speech, you will have trouble producing and internalizing the rules of phonology. Children who are deaf or hard of hearing need intensive auditory stimulation and appropriate fitting of hearing aids or cochlear implants to develop clear speech, and to develop all of the aspects of the phonology of their language system.

Essential Practice #7

> There is a difference between knowing the labels of the parts of speech (e.g., noun, verb, etc.) and having usable examples of those labels in one's vocabulary (e.g., dog, run). Children with hearing loss usually need assistance at the level of word meaning as well as word labels.

During typical language arts instruction, children learn to label the parts of speech. The job of teachers working with children who are deaf and hard of hearing is to teach both label and words. You will be teaching the meaning of different adjectives (e.g., sunny, happy, large), not just that these words are called adjectives. See Table 6.2 for some of the parts of speech that you may need to teach to deaf and hard of hearing children.

Table 6.2   Parts of Speech for Teachers in Teaching Children Who Are Deaf and Hard of Hearing

Nouns: count and mass

Verbs: transitive, intransitive, linking, and auxiliary

Pronouns, adjectives, adverbs, prepositions, and question forms

Connecting words such as conjunctions, determiners, and infinitives

Word derivations that act like other parts of speech, such as nouns that act like verbs (e.g., cook/cook, bake/baker), or adjectives that become adverbs (e.g., sweet/sweetly)

When you hear a child make a language mistake, you need to know what part of speech he is missing so you can focus on that category. For example, if the child says, "He gone come a my house," you need to know he is missing auxiliary verbs and infinitives so that you can encourage their use. You will also want to be able to intercede when he comes across these words in early reading material. For example, on the playground you might engage in a running commentary with the child about things other children are going to do, such as "He is going to swing. He is going to climb." In reading class, you can provide a model of what the sentence will sound like before he has to read it.

Essential Practice #8

Provide the child with experience understanding and using the adverbial system, which is an integral component of the ability to apply thinking skills, and which connects higher thought and language. Asking and answering adverbial types of questions is a key to higher-order thinking.

An adverbial is a word that can modify verbs, adjectives, and other adverbs. For example, in the sentence, "He hasn't gone *yet*," *yet* modifies the verb *gone*. In the sentence, "That's a *very* big diamond ring, you have!" *very* modifies the adjective *big*. Many other parts of speech make up the adverbial system. Prepositional phrases can function as modifiers of the verb. In the case of the sentence, *The squirrels played in the garden*, the phrase "in the garden" modifies "played" because it tells where the squirrel played. Nouns can function as adverbials (Marcus came *yesterday*). Adjectives can function as adverbials (I slept *late*). Adverbial clauses (She cried *when she saw that her dress was ruined*) are applied liberally to higher-level questions used by teachers to check comprehension (i.e., Why did she cry?). They also support discussion of aspects of an academic subject, be it comprehension of a reading passage, understanding of the physics behind simple machines, or the philosophical debate regarding trees falling in wildernesses. The questions that can be answered with a noun phrase (Who and What), that use an adjective for the answer (What color, What size, What shape, How many?), or that are answered by a verb (What did. . . . do?) are considered more concrete and easier. If the child is unfamiliar with the complexities of the adverbial system, she will have problems answering the higher-level comprehension questions.

Essential Practice #9

> Language beyond the early preschool years rapidly becomes very complex and includes challenging constructions that are often beyond the grasp of many young children with hearing loss unless they receive intense listening and language intervention.

Sentences can come in four varieties: simple, compound, complex, and compound-complex. A simple sentence has one subject and one predicate. A compound sentence combines two elements into one part (e.g., the boy and girl) or two whole sentences (e.g., He is happy and she is tired). Compound sentences can be combined using a *coordinating conjunction* (e.g., and, but, or) and each clause could stand alone if separated (called *independent clauses*). A complex sentence combines clauses together, but one clause is the main clause and the other clauses are *subordinate*. These clauses are connected by what are called *subordinating conjunctions* (e.g., that, while, before, why, because). The subordinate clause functions as an adjective, adverb, or pronoun to describe the main clause. The final way to combine clauses is the compound-complex sentence, which, as you can guess, has both coordinating and subordinating conjunctions connecting independent and subordinate clauses. Complex and compound sentences can wreak havoc with both language comprehension and reading comprehension.

Essential Practice #10

> Language is a very complicated topic to study. The more you learn about how children learn language, the better you will be able to teach them. Learn the rules of language yourself.

You might not believe it, but children's brains love rules. Language is controlled by rules. It is our job to understand these rules and present them to children with hearing loss so they can learn them well enough to play the communication game. There is much to learn and explore about how language works. The effective teacher will make use of the many resources available to improve his understanding of the intricacies of language and communication. Resources include textbooks, online grammar Web sites, English teachers, teachers of the deaf, and speech-language pathologists. Some print resources are listed at the end of the chapter.

How do babies learn rules? The human brain tries to find patterns in everything. The infant's and child's brains scrutinize the patterns of language. The patterns are there, and when given appropriate, meaningful stimulation, the human brain can't be stopped from organizing communication into a pattern, or mental grammar. Language develops spontaneously in the typically hearing child, without conscious effort, without formal instruction, and without an awareness of underlying organization. Language ability is distinct from more general processing of information or behaving intelligently.

People know how to talk in more or less the same [way] spiders know how to spin webs . . . because [spiders] have spider brains which give them the urge to spin and the competence to succeed. (Pinker, 1994, p. 5)

The difference between language and spider webs is that language develops in interaction with others, whereas spiders don't learn much from interactions with other spiders.

Essential Practice #11

> Human beings like to make sense of the world by making patterns and fitting things together. Language has patterns and is modular. We can fit our thoughts into the modules of language to communicate very complex ideas.

Language is modular in nature. Consider a car. If you break a light, the technician takes the whole module out and replaces it. He can put in a $25 junk yard version or a very expensive, top of the line halogen model. We do the same thing with language.

Consider the following sentences:

(1) A _____ crossed the road.

(2) My brother _____ a fence.

The first sentence leaves a slot for a noun phrase module, and the second gives you a slot for a verb phrase module. Review the following phrases/ modules. Some of these modules go with the first sentence and some with the second. Your understanding of the rules of grammar allows you to fit the correct modules into the correct slots:

- ran his bulldozer over

- dog with really big feet

- has been considering the pros and cons of putting up

- person might wonder why the chicken

Even though we speak using a string of words, one after another, the modular organization of language allows the mind to express complicated and interwoven thoughts. When teaching language to young children, they must first have the modules (i.e., noun phrases, verb phrases, adjectival phrases, and adverbial phrases). Then language becomes a process of helping them learn ever-increasingly complex components to fit into the modules. For example, if Johnny says "Daddy ball," we know that he doesn't have the verb module, so we will teach him about the use of verbs. However, if he says, "Me wanna go a baf-room," we know that he has all the modules. Our task in this instance is to change the junkyard version "me" to the halogen version "I."

Essential Practice #12

> The teacher must account for the biological, environmental, and cognitive factors that affect a child's language development. In addition, the teacher must interact conversationally in relevant ways to account for these factors.

The process of language development follows an order that is virtually the same from child to child and from culture to culture. Children developing language make similar errors during the course of development. The onset of the first word occurs at about the same age for all children. Each child passes through sensitive periods for different aspects of language as the brain structures itself. Mother Nature has set it up so that we have sensitive periods in which our brains may be more focused on developing a certain aspect of language than on the others (Newport, 1991; Ruben, 1997). The earliest sensitive period is for the development of sounds of language (phonology). The sensitive period for syntax and morphology begins after that (Grimshaw, Adelstein, Bryden, & MacKinnon, 1998; Newport, 1991). Vocabulary and semantics continue to develop all through life. Rules of syntax are especially vulnerable when delays in stimulation occur.

Although it is clear that language acquisition is biologically based, no child can acquire a language without stimulation. Language development requires interactive communication, not passive stimulation. The two necessary properties of the interactions that lead to language acquisition are *corrections* and *relevant conversational replies.* Adults tend to correct content rather than form. For example, if a child were to see a dog running and say, "Kitty ranning," the adult would more likely say, "No dear, that's a doggie not a kitty" rather than correcting the grammar. Relevant conversational replies are statements made by the adult commenting on what the child has said. For example, when the child says, "Doggie running," a relevant conversational reply could be, "Yes, and isn't he cute?" Children seem to progress more rapidly when adults comment, expand, explain, and define the world with them.

In order for the language input to lead to the child developing correct language, the input must be *processable* both semantically and structurally. Children respond best to input just above their current level of functioning (Vygotsky, 1978). If the language stimulus is too complex, it will be beyond the child's processing ability. If the stimulus is at or below the child's current language level, the child will not be receiving enough information to make progress.

Language development relies on cognitive maturation. Language makes its appearance when actions begin to be represented in thought. During the first two years of life an infant learns to discriminate herself from the rest of the world. The child learns that she has power over herself, objects, and other people in her world. There exists a close relationship between language and thought that runs throughout the language hierarchy. Thinking skills associated with different language stages were presented in the chapters on infants and toddlers, preschoolers, and children in the primary grades.

Essential Practice #13

> The child uses all the clues available to him to understand what is said to him and to incorporate new elements (e.g., words, morphemes, or phrase structure) into his language system. He accesses all that is comprehensible. If a language stimulus is not comprehensible, then he cannot incorporate it into his language system, and it must be specifically taught.

Teachers must be able to differentiate between when a structure can be developed through careful stimulation and when a structure will need to be taught directly. Understanding the continuum of typical language development and where a child with a hearing loss falls in that continuum is an important consideration when making that distinction. Knowing how much of a delay there is in your child's language level and those of his peers with normal hearing also affects the type of remediation you will choose. You should also consider the child's age, learning style, and ability to perceive speech through listening when determining the strategies that will be most successful.

Essential Practice #14

> Spoken language and thinking go hand in hand. Always work from a base of meaningful activities, focusing on the concept, or thought, as well as on speech and language. Keep the connection between thought and language foremost in your mind as you work with children who are deaf or hard of hearing.

Language and thought are mutually dependent. As language develops, our ability to share thoughts and ideas develops. Similarly, as our thoughts and ideas develop, language ability increases. In fact, language may even have a central role in shaping thought (Biever, 2004; see Figure 6.2).

Speech devoid of thought is useless. Children can learn to say phrases without understanding their meaning. Unless the words have meaning for a child, neither the language nor the thought can develop beyond a most primitive stage.

Figure 6.2   Relationship Between Language and Thought

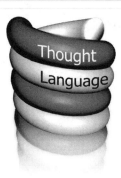

SOURCE: Illustration by James Poulakos 2006.

PHYSIOLOGICAL LEVEL: THE PHYSIOLOGY OF SPEECH

Essential Practice #15

> The unique physical aspects of the hearing and speech mechanisms in each child affect the approach you will take when helping that child learn to communicate. Each child is different from another, and you need to individualize your approaches and techniques.

The physiological process of speaking involves four components: respiration, phonation, articulation, and resonation. A speaker forms a thought from her vast array of information, and then the brain transforms thoughts into neural impulses, one of which is the impulse for *respiration.* The speaker takes in a breath, and then breathes it out, controlling the amount of breath used to support the flow of speech. When she speaks, her vocal cords (folds) usually vibrate. When the vocal folds vibrate, this is called *phonation,* or *voicing* (see Figure 6.3). Some sounds of speech are voiced (e.g., /v/, /z/) and some sounds are not voiced (e.g., /f/, /s/).

The sound is also modified through *articulation* (see Figure 6.4). The articulators include the lips, teeth, tongue, and palates. The articulators touch or come close together in different ways to form the sounds of speech. For example, the bottom lip touches the upper row of teeth for the sound /f/. As the positions of the articulators change from one speech sound to another, the shape of the vocal tract also changes.

After the breath stream passes through the vocal folds, it enters the cavities of the throat, mouth, and nose, which form the shape of the vocal tract. Resonance of speech is the pattern of vibration determined by the action of the vocal folds and shape of the vocal tract (see Figure 6.5).

The actions of respiration, phonation, resonance, and articulation combine to form the sounds that leave a person's mouth and pass through the air.

Figure 6.3   Phonation

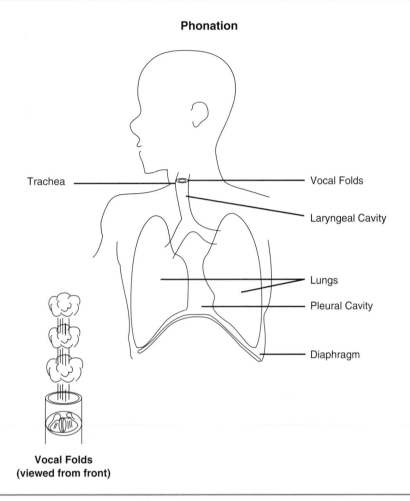

Phonation

Trachea

Vocal Folds

Laryngeal Cavity

Lungs

Pleural Cavity

Diaphragm

**Vocal Folds
(viewed from front)**

SOURCE: Illustration by James Poulakos 2006.

Figure 6.4   Articulation

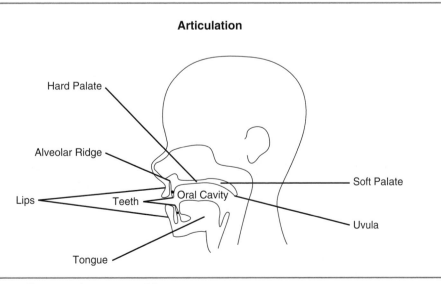

Articulation

Hard Palate

Alveolar Ridge

Soft Palate

Lips

Teeth   Oral Cavity

Uvula

Tongue

SOURCE: Illustration by James Poulakos 2006.

Figure 6.5 Resonation

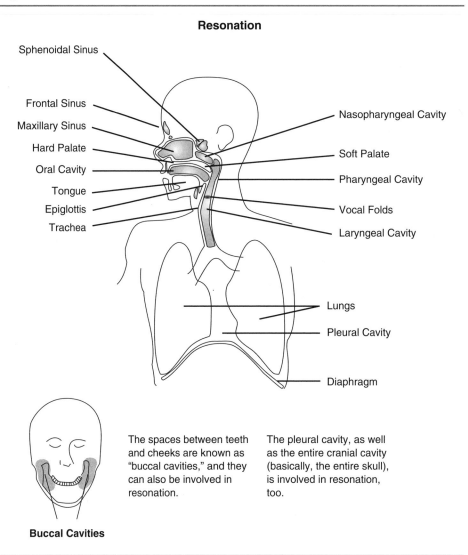

Resonation

Sphenoidal Sinus

Frontal Sinus
Maxillary Sinus
Hard Palate
Oral Cavity
Tongue
Epiglottis
Trachea

Nasopharyngeal Cavity

Soft Palate
Pharyngeal Cavity
Vocal Folds
Laryngeal Cavity

Lungs
Pleural Cavity

Diaphragm

The spaces between teeth and cheeks are known as "buccal cavities," and they can also be involved in resonation.

The pleural cavity, as well as the entire cranial cavity (basically, the entire skull), is involved in resonation, too.

Buccal Cavities

SOURCE: Illustration by James Poulakos 2006.

We call this the *speech signal.* If a young person has malformations of the speech structures or has physiological problems with respiration, phonation, or articulation, then it will be a greater challenge for this child to learn to speak.

PHYSIOLOGICAL LEVEL: THE PHYSIOLOGY OF HEARING

The ear is made up of three main sections: the outer ear, the middle ear, and the inner ear. The outer ear and middle ear: (a) collect the acoustical sound pressure energy; (b) transform acoustic energy to physical vibration and movement; and (c) amplify and focus that energy, making it strong enough to stimulate the sensory cells in the inner ear. The sensory cells in the inner ear respond to the vibration and fire the neural impulses, which excite the auditory nerve. The auditory nerve carries impulses from the inner ear to the auditory cortex in the brain.

Figure 6.6   Schematic of the Outer, Middle, and Inner Ear With Auditory Nerve

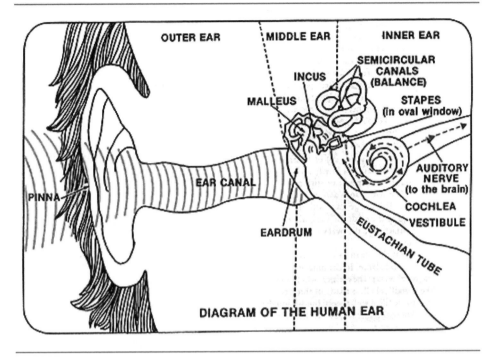

SOURCE: Used with permission of Gallaudet University.

The Outer Ear

One part of the outer ear is called the *pinna.* The pinna serves as a collector of sounds, something like a scoop, with the folds in the pinna funneling the sound into the ear canal. When someone is talking too quietly, you can scoop up more sound by cupping your hand behind your ear and channeling sound into the *ear canal* (see Figure 6.6).

The Middle Ear

The ear canal leads to the eardrum, or *tympanic membrane,* which is the demarcation between the outer and middle ear. On the other side of the tympanic membrane there is an open, air-filled space in the skull, called the *middle ear cavity.* There are three small bones in the middle ear. The first is called the *malleus* and is attached to the back of the tympanic membrane. The malleus has a muscle called the *tensor tympanus* attached to it, connecting it to the wall of the middle ear. The tensor tympanus pulls on the malleus, stiffening the tympanic membrane as a reflex in response to loud noises. Some hearing evaluations measure this reflex; we call this *acoustic reflex testing.* The back and forth movement of the tympanic membrane pushes and pulls on the malleus, causing the bone attached to it, the *incus* or anvil, to move. The incus is connected to the third bone in the chain, the *stapes* or stirrup. The end of the stapes fits into the inner ear, pushing in and out of the inner ear, causing the liquid in the inner ear to move along with the vibration of the bones.

The middle ear is connected to the back of the throat by the *Eustachian tube.* The Eustachian tube allows air pressure changes on one side of the tympanic membrane (outside the head) to be equalized on the other side (inside the head). When you yawn, you open the back of your throat at the Eustachian tube, allowing the air pressure to enter into your middle ear and equalize with the pressure in the air around you. Then your tympanic membrane goes back to its normal position. You may not hear as well when your tympanic membrane is being pulled or pushed by air pressure changes.

The Inner Ear

The cochlea is a small bony spiral shaped like a conch shell, which contains the inner ear mechanisms. The cochlea is filled with a fluid similar to cerebrospinal fluid. The cochlea is connected to the semi-circular canals (which give the brain information about balance and orientation in space) and shares the same fluid. If you were to unroll the cochlea, you'd see that there is a bony shelf and membrane running down the middle dividing the cochlea into a top half and a bottom half. The basal end (closest to the middle ear) of the cochlea has two openings. The opening on top is called the *oval window.* This is where the middle ear bone, the stapes, fits into the cochlea and where the stapes pushes and pulls to vibrate the fluid in the cochlea. The opening on the bottom of the base of the cochlea is called the round window and is covered by a membrane. It moves back and forth in response to the vibrations in the fluid. This response allows the vibration to travel all the way along the length of the cochlea (see Figure 6.7).

The bony shelf and membrane in the middle of the cochlea hold the *organ of Corti,* the sense organ for sound. The organ of Corti contains hair cells lined up under an overhanging membrane called the *tectorial membrane.* The top of each hair cell has filaments, called *cilia,* which brush against the bottom of the tectorial membrane. The bottom of each hair cell connects to the auditory nerve that runs along the length of the cochlea. The vibration of the liquid in the cochlea causes the tectorial membrane to move. If there is enough movement, the hair cells stimulate the auditory nerve endings to fire. The auditory nerve carries the signal to the brain. The normal cochlea is sensitive to a wide range of intensities and frequencies of sound.

A hearing loss can be caused by many different problems. The bones of the middle ear can be malformed or missing. The middle ear can be filled with fluid or tissue. The hair cells of the organ of Corti can be damaged or missing. The fluid in the inner ear could be affected by leaks (called "fistulas"). The structure of the cochlea could be weak and deteriorating over time (e.g., enlarged vestibular aqueducts). The flow of the fluid through the inner ear could be disturbed through malformations in the channels that carry the fluid (e.g., Connexin 26 mutation). The cochlea can have fewer than two and one-half turns (called "Mondini's defect"), even to the extent that there are no turns at all (called "common cavity Mondini's defect"). In come cases there is no cochlea at all.

ACOUSTIC LEVEL

You will note on the speech chain that a spoken sound can go in two directions: through the air to a listener and through the air back to the speaker. As we talk, we hear ourselves. This sets up a *feedback loop* through which we are constantly

Figure 6.7   Views of the Cochlea: (a) A Longitudinal Section of the Unrolled
Cochlea; (b) A Cross-Section Through the Unrolled Cochlea

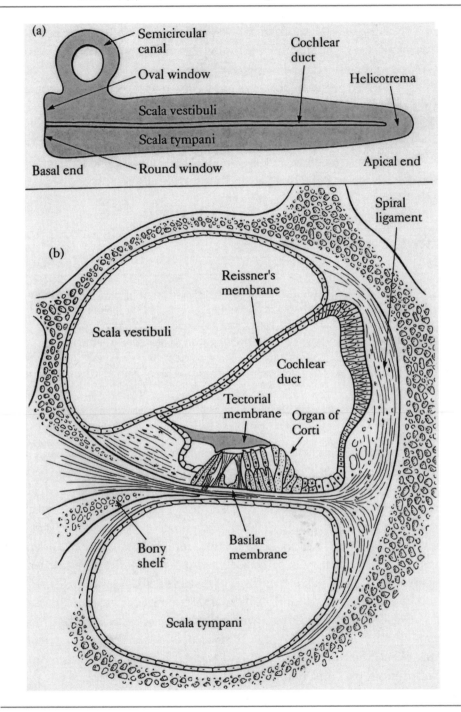

SOURCE: From *The Speech Chain: The Physics and Biology of Spoken Language* by Peter B. Denes and
Elliott N. Pinson, copyright © 1993 by W. H. Freeman and Company. Reprinted by permission of
Henry Holt and Company, LLC.

comparing what we hear ourselves say with what we intended to say. This feedback loop is a very important feature of the language development process
because children speak the way they hear (Pollack, Goldberg, & Caleffe-Schenck,
1997). The *auditory feedback loop* is also a necessary precursor to babbling

(Koopmans-van Beinum, Clement, & van den Dikkenberg-Pot, 2001). We can get a pretty good idea of what a child can hear by what he can say. The better the technology we use (i.e., hearing aids, cochlear implants, and other listening devices), the better signal the child will get, and so his speech will be better. The more carefully we provide sounds so the child can listen to himself compare what he has said with what he is supposed to say, the easier it will be for him to learn to speak. We hear with our ears, but *we listen with our brains*. Learning to listen makes learning to talk a lot easier. We must engage our brains to listen to and think about sounds. This is why we use the term *auditory brain development* to describe the processes children go through as they learn to listen and speak. Another term we use when we talk about auditory brain development is *auditory perceptual development*. Refer to Chapter 1 for further discussion on the auditory feedback loop.

Essential Practice #16

> There is a direct link between what a child hears and what he says. Understanding the relationship between the acoustic (sound) properties of speech and a child's level of hearing (as shown on an audiogram) will help you target stimulation to the individual child's listening needs. The audiogram will also indicate the type of loss. Consult the child's aided audiogram (i.e., what he hears with his hearing aid and/or cochlear implant) to help determine appropriate instructional objectives and procedures.

There are three aspects to the speech signal: frequency, intensity, and duration (Fry, 1999). *Frequency* refers to how many cycles of a sound wave occur in a time frame (usually one second). Our brains perceive frequency as pitch. The pitch of a sound can be high, like a bird's singing, or low, like the rumble of thunder. The measure of how many cycles of a wave occur in one second is defined by the term, Hertz (Hz). *Intensity* is the strength (amplitude) or amount of energy in a sound wave. Intensity is perceived as loudness. We describe intensity by sound pressure level, which is measured in decibels (dB). A low amplitude wave is heard as a soft or quiet sound. A high amplitude wave causes a loud sound. The *duration* of sound is measured in seconds, milliseconds, and in even finer distinctions of time. Duration is an important component of early pattern recognition and should be the first place we start when helping a child to listen and speak. Our brain uses duration cues to interpret different aspects of the speech signal including syllable accent and short versus long vowel distinctions.

Essential Practice #17

> Teachers need to have an understanding of a child's audiogram and what it means in relation to what the child will be able to hear in the classroom.

An *audiogram* is a graphic representation of an individual's pattern of hearing. Figure 6.8 is an example of an audiogram a teacher might receive. An audiogram has two very important characteristics. The lines going vertically represent the frequency or pitch of a sound. Marks on the left side of the audiogram refer to low-frequency sounds. Marks on the right side of the audiogram refer to high-frequency sounds. The lines going horizontally represent the decibel level or loudness of a sound. A mark at the bottom of a page tells us that a sound has to be very loud before a child will hear it. A mark at the top of the page tells us that a sound can be very soft and a child will hear it.

An audiologist conducts *pure-tone testing* of the individual frequencies to determine the loudness level at which the child can just barely hear or detect each frequency. The level at which the child barely detects sound is called the *threshold.* Pure-tone testing is initially done with the child not wearing hearing

Figure 6.8   Comprehensive Audiogram

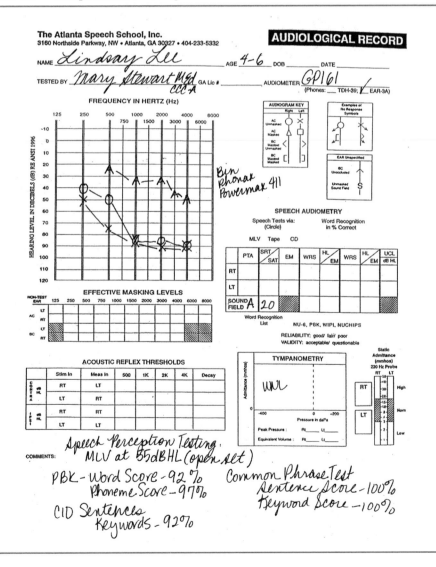

aids. This is called *unaided testing.* The audiologist measures the child's hearing at the different pitches and makes marks on a graph, noting the decibel level and the pitch. The results from the child's right ear will be marked with a circle (sometimes using red ink) and the left ear will be marked with an X (sometimes using blue ink). The audiologist connects these markings for each ear with a line. The audiologist will also mark an "A" on an audiogram to indicate testing done with the child wearing her hearing aid, or *aided testing.* A child's pattern of pure-tone thresholds across a range of tones is called his *acuity.* The audiologist may calculate a *pure-tone average* (PTA), which is an average of the pure-tone threshold values at 500, 1,000 Hz, and 2,000 Hz. Typically each ear will have a different pattern of response. The audiogram form itself will have a key explaining the various other marks you may see. In the example given, we know that Lindsay, who has a PTA of about 42 dB, has slightly better hearing in her right ear than her left in the lower frequencies.

Audiologists gather information in different manners. In *behavioral response testing,* the audiologist will look for reactions to sound such as body movements and changes in facial expression. In *visual response testing,* the child responds to sound by looking at a stimulus that appears only after a sound has been presented. For example, the child may be trained (i.e., conditioned) to look at a video screen after he has heard a sound. In *play audiometry,* the child makes an overt, observable response to a stimulus, such as putting a peg in a board when she hears a sound. Audiologists also use different stimuli for gathering pure-tone testing results. In *air conduction testing,* a sound is presented to the child through the air using speakers in the audiology booth (called *soundfield testing*), through earphone inserts placed in the child's ear canal, or through headphones placed over the child's outer ear. Lindsay was tested through soundfield testing on one of the tests given. In *bone conduction testing,* the sound is presented through a bone vibrator, or *oscillator* that vibrates in response to sound. The oscillator is placed directly on the child's head, usually on the bony projection just behind the pinna. In the case of bone conduction testing, by placing the oscillator on the child's skull, the vibration is presented directly to the inner ear, bypassing the outer ear and the middle ear.

Evaluations should be conducted by a professional audiologist who is certified by the American Board of Audiology and has one of the following groups of initials after his or her name: "F-AAA" (Fellow—American Academy of Audiology), "CCC-A" (Certificate of Clinical Competence—Audiologist), or "CF-A" (Clinical Fellow—Audiologist). All audiologists have either a doctorate in Audiology (AuD, PhD) or a master's degree. Evaluations from a hearing aid dealer who is not also an audiologist may not contain the necessary depth and breadth of information you will need.

Through analysis of the results of all tests given, the audiologist determines the type of loss a child has. A loss might be *conductive, sensorineural,* or it might be referred to as *auditory dyssynchrony* (sometimes called auditory neuropathy). In a conductive loss, the part of the ear that "conducts" the sound to the inner ear has one or more problems. In a sensorineural loss, the neural system that transmits the sound to the brain malfunctions. Auditory dyssynchrony is a condition in which the outer hair cells of the cochlea are normal but there is a problem with neural transmission to the brain. In other instances, the audiologist may determine from the testing that a combination of factors has caused a *mixed* hearing loss. Table 6.3 identifies additional testing that might be conducted.

See Resource B for commonly used speech intelligibility tests. Always remember that speech testing requires that the child knows the words being presented to him. (An exception to this rule is the speech awareness threshold.) It is inappropriate to perform these speech tasks on a young child who doesn't have the vocabulary necessary to respond correctly. When an audiologist is fitting a hearing aid, he or she wants to make note of the child's dynamic range. The

Table 6.3   Additional Tests of Hearing

Type	Description
Visual Inspection	Examination of the outer ear, ear canal, and eardrum (tympanic membrane). The audiologist uses an instrument called an *otoscope* to examine the ear canal and the tympanic membrane for any type of malformation, obstruction, or indication of infection that will affect the child's hearing.
Tympanometry	Measurement of the movement of the tympanic membrane. The audiologist inserts a small tube into the child's ear canal, and the tympanometer increases and decreases the air pressure in the ear canal slightly. The tympanometer then measures whether the tympanic membrane responds normally to these changes. The results of this evaluation are printed out in graph form called a *tympanogram*.
Oto-Acoustic Emissions	Measurement of the inner ear's perception of sound
Acoustic Reflex	Measurement of reflexive activation of the tensor tympani muscle in the middle ear in response to a sound
Auditory Brainstem Response	Measurement of the brainstem's neural response to sound
Speech Awareness Threshold	Measurement of how loud a word must be before a child responds to it
Speech Reception Threshold	Measurement of how loud speech has to be in order for a child to repeat 50 percent of a word list correctly or point to pictures of words spoken through a loudspeaker
Desired Sensation Level (DSL)	Computer-assisted method of determining the appropriate fit of the hearing aid, based on setting the hearing aid to amplify sound correctly between the child's threshold and uncomfortable loudness level
Speech Intelligibility Testing	Measurement of the child's ability to discriminate or recognize speech. This is usually done at supra-threshold levels, or levels clearly above the child's threshold. The audiologist uses specific words, phrases, or sentences. In *closed-set testing*, the child has the advantage of knowing what possible words she will hear. In *open-set testing*, the child has to repeat a word, phrase, or sentence or respond to a question with no prior knowledge of content.

dynamic range is the difference between the softest sound a person can perceive (the threshold) and the loudest sound a person can stand before it is uncomfortable (called the *uncomfortable loudness level* or UCL). Everything we hear without discomfort occurs within the dynamic range. The greater the hearing loss, the narrower the dynamic range. The narrower the dynamic range, the greater difficulty a child will have perceiving differences among sounds (see Figure 6.9).

Figure 6.9 Audiogram of Dynamic Range

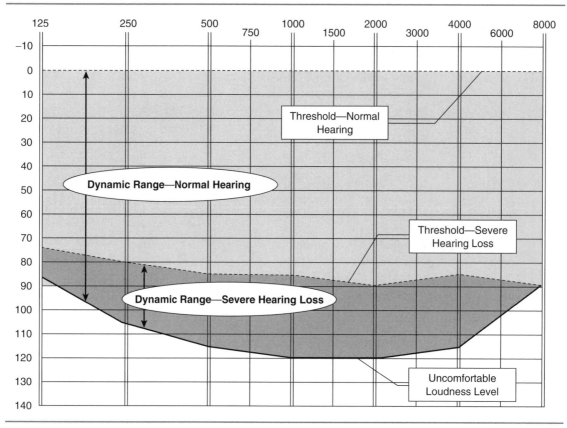

SOURCE: Courtesy of Ellen Estes.

Essential Practice #18

> When helping a child learn to listen to speech, always present sounds that have noticeable differences. This is necessary so the child can learn to discriminate one sound from another. If we don't make sounds noticeably different, the child will merely be guessing at the differences.

An important way that we know we are providing a noticeable difference is to analyze the acoustic features of a speech sound, in particular, the formants of the sounds. This analysis tells us which part of a sound the child can hear and which he cannot.

Say the vowel -oo- as in shoe. You will feel a vibration in your vocal tract. The rate at which your vocal folds open and close is called the *fundamental frequency* (F0). It provides the lowest energy, or frequency, to a sound. The sound produced by the vocal folds has other, higher frequencies, called *harmonics* (a.k.a. overtones). These harmonics are amplified (made louder) or damped (made quieter) by the shape of your vocal tract. The amplified harmonics are called *formants* (F1, F2, F3, etc). As a person speaks, the shape of the vocal tract changes. The different shapes amplify different formant frequencies. A person needs to perceive at least the first two formants (F1 and F2) of a sound to be able to discriminate and recognize that sound in speech.

A *spectrogram* is a visual representation of the frequency patterns of sounds. In Figure 6.10, you see a spectrogram of the sounds -ee- as in feet, -i- as in hit, -e- as in get, and -a- as in cat. The horizontal axis represents time. The vertical axis represents frequency or pitch. The intensity of a sound is shown by the darkness of a tracing. You can see the dark band of energy occurring at the first formant (F1) and a second burst of energy occurring at the second formant (F2). If you say these four sounds you will feel the differences in your

Figure 6.10 Spectrogram of Four Vowels

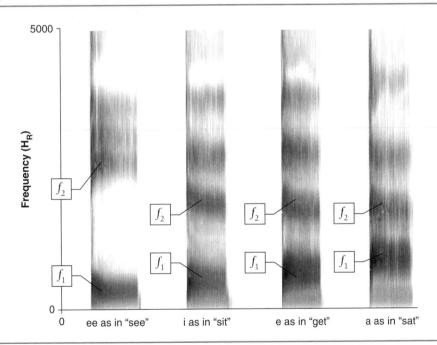

mouth. As the formants get higher, their intensity (loudness) tends to get lower, as seen by the gradually lighter tracings.

Figure 6.11 shows the first and second formants of some vowels of English. In this figure, frequency is shown on the horizontal axis (unlike Figure 6.10). While there is some variation from speaker to speaker and between men and women, we all produce vowels with similar energy patterns (De Boysson-Bardie, 1989). The squares on the left labeled f_1 represent the first formants, and the tipped squares on the right labeled f_2 represent the second formants. The vowels toward the bottom have high-frequency second formants. A child who does not have sufficient hearing above 1,000 Hz may have trouble distinguishing one vowel sound from another. Never expect a child to hear the differences between sounds he cannot hear. If we develop auditory goals outside the child's capacity to hear, then the child will learn to guess at the differences between sounds rather than depend on his auditory ability (Pollack, Goldberg, & Caleffe-Schenck, 1997). Guessing is counterproductive in the beginning stages of auditory development. Fortunately the vowels -oo- and -ee- are more easily identified by adding lipreading, and the child will benefit from hearing and seeing the sound at the same time.

Figure 6.11 Formants of Some Vowels of English

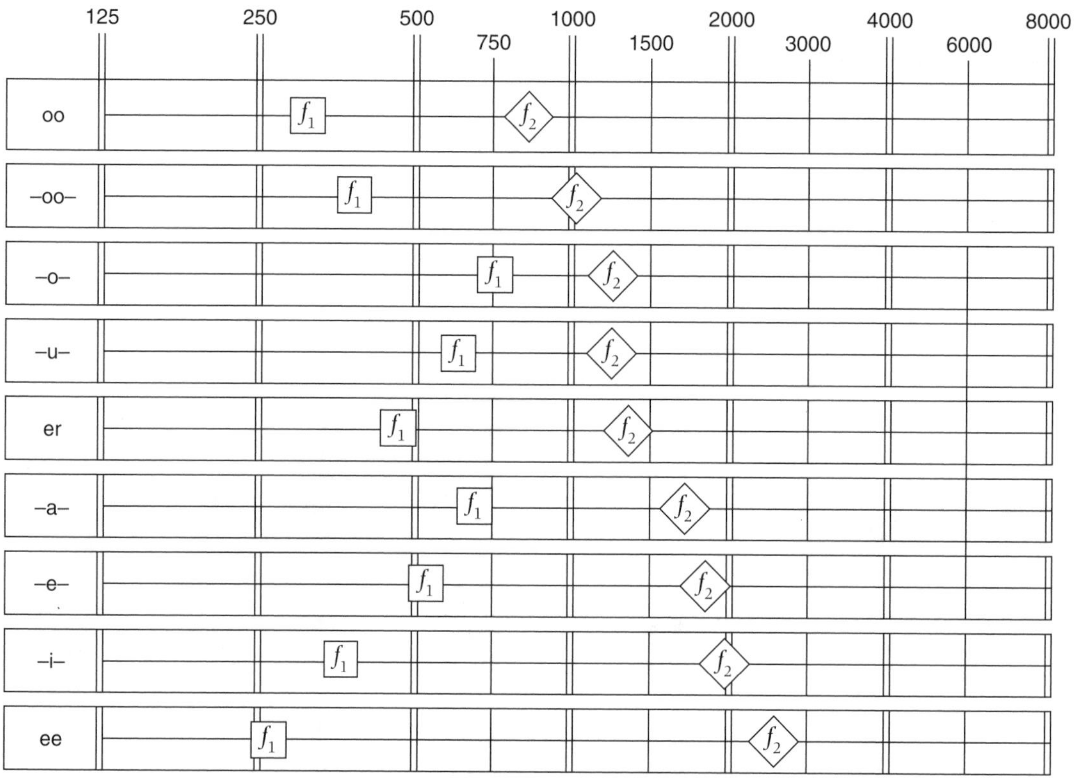

SOURCES: Courtesy of Ellen Estes based on *The Speech Chain* (Denes & Pinson, 1993); De Boysson-Bardie (1989).

Essential Practice #19

Always teach new speech skills in coarticulation (i.e., vowel and consonant combined) so the child can hear information from the transitions between sounds.

The brain uses the information from the vowel transition to help it understand the consonant. Speech is not static; the brain uses the transitions that occur when moving from one sound to another. The brain uses the movement from one sound to another as much as it does the sounds themselves to decode what it is hearing. Look at the spectrogram of a person speaking the word "see," and then the word, "she" (Figure 6.12). You can see that the first sound (/s/) has a high-frequency component (Location 1= L1). Now look at the place where the speaker's voice moves from the high /s/ sound to the vowel sound (-ee-; Location 2 = L2). We call this the second formant transition or the point of transition where the energy slopes into the next formant band.

In the word "she," the *sh-* sound is composed of a narrower range of frequencies (Location 3 = L3). The *sh-* sound also has a lower second formant than the /s/ as you can see by the tracings (Location 4 = L4), and it transitions differently into the *–ee-* sound (Location 5 = L5). Your brain uses information from transitions to help perceive "see" and "she." In other words, the brain uses both steady-state frequency and transition information to decode what it hears. For this reason it is extremely important to teach each speech sound in the context of other sounds. This is called coarticulation (Denes & Pinson, 1993; Ling, 2002).

Figure 6.12 Spectrogram of Speech Transition Points

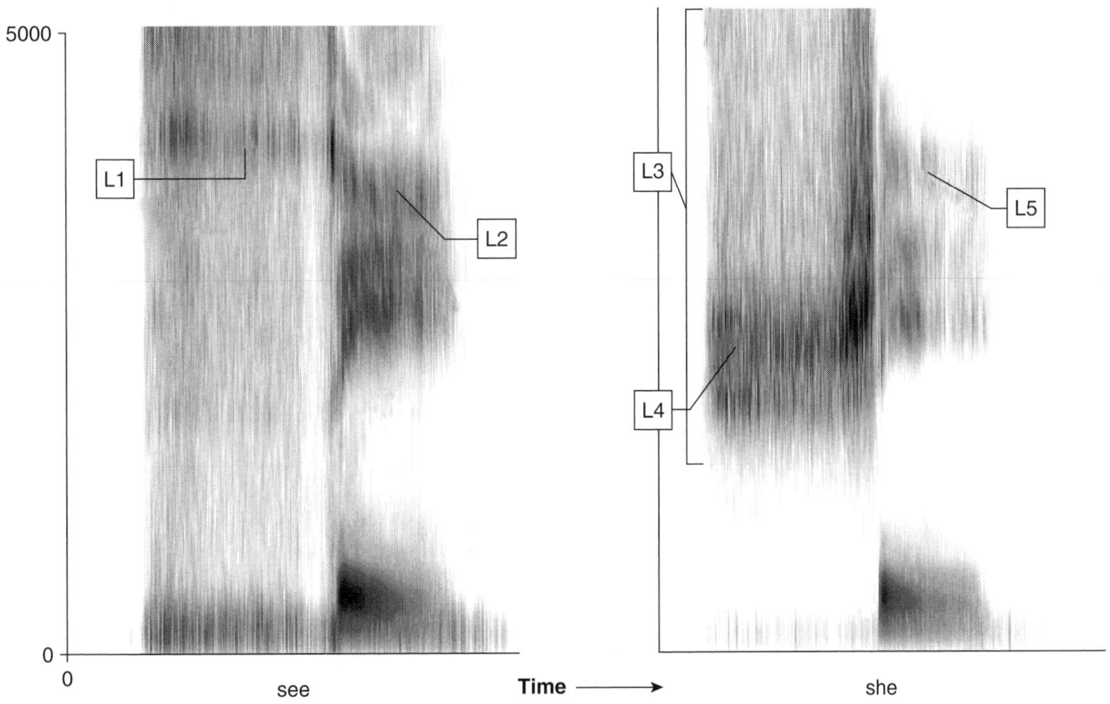

SOURCE: Illustration by James Poulakos and Ellen Estes 2006.

Essential Practice #20

> Speaking in close range to the child's hearing aids is most important when teaching the lowest and highest frequency sounds.

As described in the previous section on testing, the fine line between hearing something that is very soft or not hearing it is called the *threshold of hearing*

(Berg & Stork, 1995). There is a large range between the softest sounds of speech and the loudest sounds of speech. Many aspects of speech fall outside the average intensity range of speech (50–65 dB). Sounds at the lower frequencies and the higher frequencies are quieter than sounds in the middle of the spectrum. Vowels are the strongest (loudest) sounds of speech. Vowels are classified as open and closed. *Open vowels* are formed with the tongue in position away from the roof of the mouth to allow the air to flow through. *Closed vowels* are formed with the tongue close to the roof of the mouth to constrict the flow of air. Closed vowels are quieter than open vowels. The strongest vowel sound is the open vowel, -aw, which is three times stronger than the weakest (softest) vowel sound, the closed vowel -ee-. Consonants also have a range of loudness. The /r/ sound as in rug, is the strongest consonant and has about the same intensity as the weakest vowel sound. The /r/ sound is 200 times stronger than the voiceless /th/ (as in "thing"). Nasal formants are weaker than vowel formants (see Table 6.4).

Table 6.4   Strong and Weak Speech Sounds

Strong Sounds	Description
aw	(strongest, or loudest vowel)
central vowels	(next loudest)
r	(strongest consonant)

Weak Sounds	Description
ee	(weakest vowel)
voiceless th	(weakest consonant)
vowel formants	
voiced/voiceless fricative turbulence	

SOURCES: Denes and Pinson (1993); Clarke School for the Deaf (1995).

Essential Practice #21

> Talk closer to the child's ear. Don't talk louder.

The way to increase intensity when speaking is to get closer to the child, not to speak louder. When you speak louder, you change the acoustic properties of your speech so the child is not listening to the typical sound patterns. If the child cannot hear speech at three feet, move closer. Normal speech at three feet is around 50–65 dB, and that same normal speech at three inches is 90 dB. This is important to remember when helping a child learn to listen. Figure 6.13 shows a graph of the percentages of words that people correctly identified when an examiner spoke the words to them at different loudness levels. This figure demonstrates that if something is very quiet, then most people identify only a few or none of the words correctly. It is not until words are about 60 dB that most people identify most of the words correctly. The implication for the child whose threshold for hearing is at 30 dB, for example, is that he will miss many of the words he hears, even though he is aware of them. Getting closer to the child will improve the chances to perceive a sound.

Figure 6.13 Understanding at Different Loudness Levels

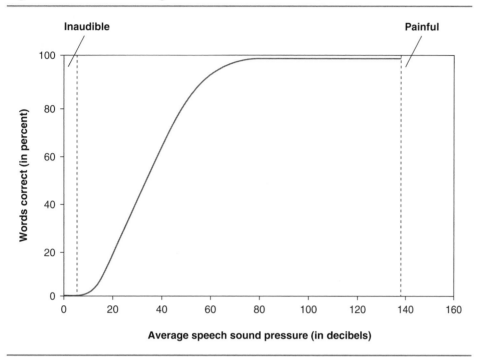

SOURCE: From *The Speech Chain: The Physics and Biology of Spoken Language* by Peter B. Denes and Elliott N. Pinson, copyright © 1993 by W. H. Freeman and Company. Reprinted by permission of Henry Holt and Company, LLC.

Essential Practice #22

Children need to practice hearing and using speech with varied duration.

The brain uses duration of a sound more than relative loudness to interpret a word. For example, when you lengthen the first syllable of the word OBject as opposed to the second syllable, obJECT, the meaning changes. Duration is a controlling factor.

Essential Practice #23

When asking a child to discriminate between two sounds, always make sure that the differences between the sounds are far enough apart for his brain to perceive.

How far apart do two things (sights, sounds, odors, tastes, touches) have to be in order for us to notice they are different? In any aspect of sensation (seeing, hearing, smelling, tasting, feeling), a *minimal difference* is required in order to produce a *just noticeable difference* (Denes & Pinson, 1993). A child with a hearing loss requires a larger minimal difference to perceive just noticeable differences in frequency and intensity. This not the case for duration. The critical difference for duration is virtually the same for people with normal hearing and people with hearing loss. This is why we begin auditory stimulation by helping children listen to different durations of sounds (e.g., "ahhhhhh" for an airplane versus "hop" for a rabbit). When we work on frequency or intensity differences, the child needs to master larger, more noticeable changes first (e.g., "Mom" versus "see"), and smaller differences later (e.g., "bee" versus "me").

While Figure 6.13 shows the percentage of words people can hear at different loudness levels, Figure 6.14 helps demonstrate the sounds that are lost when there is little or no hearing at different frequency levels.

Figure 6.14 Audiogram of Speech Sounds

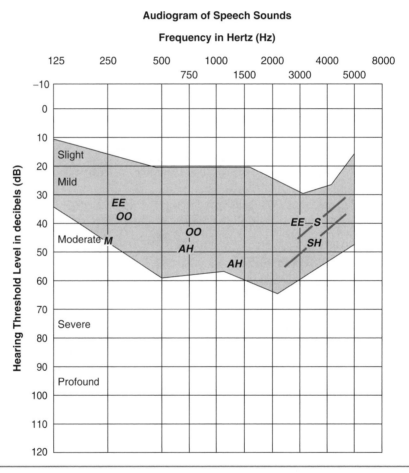

SOURCE: Customized by Brad Ingrao, Electronic Deaf Education Network.

HEARING AIDS, COCHLEAR IMPLANTS, AND ASSISTIVE LISTENING DEVICES

Essential Practice #24

> Careful, ongoing monitoring of a listening device and the auditory environment improve the chances that a child will make progress in listening and understanding sounds.

There are many devices available today to help deliver sound to a child with a hearing loss (see Figure 6.15). An audiologist programs or tunes a child's hearing aid or cochlear implant to stimulate the ear at the most appropriate levels based on the child's individual needs as identified in the audiological assessment.

Figure 6.15 Various Listening Devices

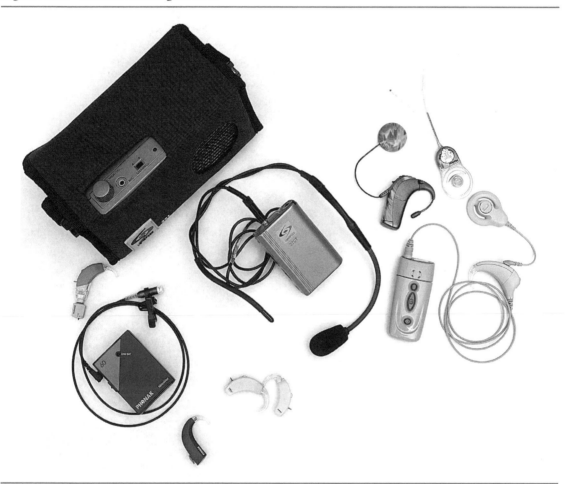

SOURCE: Photographed by John Zimmermann.

Hearing Aids

The purpose of a hearing aid is to make sound louder. There are different types of hearing aids; each has a different size and configuration. All hearing aids use batteries. They also have microphones that pick up sound, electronic circuits that process sound and make it louder, and speakers that emit this louder sound. In all hearing aids, sound travels down a tube through material specifically fitted to the child's ear and into the ear canal. The material that fits into the child's ear is called an *earmold*. A snug fit between the earmold and canal is very important. If the fit is not snug, sound will leak out from the end of the earmold and will be picked up by the hearing aid's own microphone, creating *feedback*. Feedback from a hearing aid sounds like a high-pitched squeal. If a hearing aid is continually feeding back, it is important to check whether there is a crack in the earmold or the tubing, or whether the child needs a new earmold because his ears have grown and the earmold no longer fits snugly. The audiologist can assist in determining the cause of the feedback and in making a new earmold, if necessary.

Cochlear Implants

For some hearing losses, merely making the sound louder is not enough; loudness alone does not make a sound clear and does not make speech understandable. In these cases, the fidelity of the sound that is delivered to the brain is not clear. The sensation is similar to listening to a radio station that is just out of reach of the antenna. The speech becomes garbled and interspersed with static. Even if you turn up the volume on your radio, you have a hard time understanding what the announcer is saying. When this is the case, children and adults often benefit from receiving a cochlear implant.

Every cochlear implant has an internal device and an external device. The internal device is composed of an electrode array attached to a receiver. The electrode array is surgically inserted into the cochlea and the receiver is placed under the skin of the scalp somewhere above and/or behind the pinna. The external device has a microphone, a sound processing computer, a transmitter, and batteries. At least one electric cord connects the various components of the external device.

The microphone picks up sound and sends it to the sound processor. The sound processor analyzes the sound, transforms it into electrical energy, and sends it through the transmitter to the internal device. The internal device sends the electronic coding to the electrode array that has been inserted into the cochlea. The electrodes directly stimulate the auditory nerve in the cochlea with electrical energy. The auditory nerve responds to the stimulation by firing and carrying the signal along the neural pathways to the auditory cortex of the brain.

The determination of whether a hearing aid or a cochlear implant is the better choice for a particular child depends on many factors. The audiologist will investigate this possibility in conjunction with the child's physician. Teachers and parents provide valuable insight into this investigation by stimulating the child throughout the day and noting his responses to various sounds.

Assistive Listening Devices

In addition to hearing aids and cochlear implants, a wide array of assistive listening devices is available. We address these under the section on managing the noise in classrooms.

Device Troubleshooting

When a device is not working, the most common cause is a dead battery. Be sure you have a supply of batteries on hand that fit the device. If the device has parts connected by a wire (or *cord*), have an extra set of cords so you can replace them quickly. Be sure you know the proper settings for the device and how to change the settings back to the right ones. Another chronic problem especially in warm climate areas is moisture from sweat. You can purchase a kit that will dry the hearing aid(s) or cochlear implant(s). When the earmold is loose, you will experience feedback. Make sure that the earmold is the correct size for the child by consulting with the audiologist. Report to the audiologist immediately any scratchy sounds or sounds that are diminished in quality. For information on troubleshooting problems with specific hearing aids and cochlear implants, consult the manufacturer's Web site or the child's audiologist. Every device comes with a troubleshooting guide that will help you quickly determine the most likely cause and solution for any problems that arise.

What to Ask and Tell the Audiologist

The Audiologist's Feedback Form (Figure 6.16) can be used to request feedback when the student goes for a visit. The audiologist will provide you with valuable information about the child's auditory potential. Keep track of the proper function of the device and your child's auditory ability, and share this information with the audiologist. Keep the child's audiologist's contact information handy in case a device needs to be returned for repair.

CLASSROOM ACOUSTICS—INCREASING THE CHILD'S ABILITY TO HEAR AND UNDERSTAND THE TEACHER AND PEERS

Essential Practice #25

> Children with normal hearing are able to block out unwanted background noises; children with hearing losses have difficulty doing this. Care must be taken to reduce background noise to the maximum extent possible, especially in the classroom, where noise coming through a hearing aid or cochlear implant can easily drown out the teacher's voice.

The noise and distance in the classroom affects how well a child can listen and perceive and understand what others are saying. Listening devices improve hearing, but other factors can make a child's challenge easier or relatively harder. Of particular importance is the child's ability to hear and understand the teacher's voice. The physical aspects that affect understanding are reverberation, signal-to-noise ratio, and distance.

The first physical aspect that affects understanding in the classroom is *reverberation*, or echo. When sound strikes a surface, it can pass through the surface, be absorbed, bounce off into a new direction, or scatter into multiple directions. Any combination of these four actions can happen at the same time. For example, the wall can absorb some of the sound and some of the sound can reflect off the wall. A hard, smooth surface tends to reflect more sound. A textured, soft surface absorbs sound. Reverberation is the sound reflecting off a surface. Reverberation adds unwanted background noise.

Figure 6.16 Audiologist's Feedback Form

AUDIOLOGIST'S FEEDBACK FORM

(Please fax or mail to school or send with parent)

_____ was seen in our office on _____.
         (Child's Name)   (Date)

<u>Type of device:</u>

____ Ear ____ Hearing Aid   Manufacturer _____   Type _____

____ Ear ____ Cochlear Implant   Manufacturer _____   Implant Type _____

                                                           Processor Type _____

<u>The following occurred:</u>

_____ Aided and/or unaided testing was done. A copy is attached.

_____ The program/settings were changed. A copy is attached.

_____ No changes were made to the fitting.

_____ Other:

<u>The following equipment changes were made:</u>

_____ Earmold impression taken   _____ New mold fitted

_____ Aid repair (Serial # _____)   _____ Loaner aid fitted

<u>Recommended settings (hearing aids):</u>

<u>Ear</u>	<u>Volume</u>	<u>Output</u>	<u>Tone</u>	<u>Other</u>
Right	_____	_____	_____	_____
Left	_____	_____	_____	_____

<u>Recommended settings (cochlear implant):</u>

Ear: ___ R; ___ L; ___ Both

SETTINGS	PROGRAM 1	PROGRAM 2	PROGRAM 3	PROGRAM 4
Strategy				
Volume				
Sensitivity				
Used for:				
Comments:				
Recommended for School:				

Comments/Specific Recommendations: _____

_____

_____

_____
           Audiologist

Phone:

Fax:

E-mail:

SOURCE: Adapted from Koch, M. E.: _Performance based trouble shooting of cochlear implants:_ AAA Convention 2002; Atlanta Speech School _Dispensing Audiologist Update_, 2006; Moog Center for Deaf Education _Team Tracking Form_, 2004.

The second physical aspect that affects understanding in the classroom is *signal-to-noise* (S/N) ratio. Transmission of a sound through a wall from an adjoining room is another source of unwanted sound in a classroom. Typically the higher frequency components of the sound are absorbed by the surface and the lower frequency components are transmitted through the wall. Other sources of background noise are mechanical devices such as air conditioning units, buzzing from florescent lights, fan sounds from projectors, paper rustling, and chair scraping to name a few. Background noises often overwhelm the teacher's voice and the voices of the other children in the room. To calculate the understandability of speech in the presence of background noise we measure the *signal-to-noise ratio* (S/N). The sound level of the background noise is subtracted from the sound level of the teacher's voice, resulting in a positive or negative number. The more positive the number, the more teacher's voice can be heard. If the S/N is a negative number, this means that the background noise is louder than the teacher's voice. An S/N of +10 is considered minimally appropriate for a classroom of children with normal hearing. Children with hearing losses require an S/N of at least +15.

A hard surface such as a marker board behind the teacher will reflect her voice into the classroom. A hard surface in the middle of a ceiling can reflect the sound to the back of the room. Some reflective surfaces strategically placed can be beneficial for speech understanding. Placing absorbent materials on the surfaces opposite to the reflective surface and on the side and rear walls and floors eliminates reverberation. For suggestions on how to manage the noise in a classroom, see Table 6.5.

Table 6.5   Managing Noise in the Classroom

Problem	Solution	Examples
Reverberation Time	Reduce the volume of the room	Lower ceilings
	Increase the sound absorption	Add "soft" materials: • Fabric-faced wall panels • Carpet • Acoustical ceiling tiles • Hanging baffles and banners • Drapes Place diffusing element on the rear wall Place convex diffusing panels throughout the room
	Splay walls out of parallel	
	Angle sections of the ceiling to spread reflection	
Mechanical Noise	Update heating, ventilation and air conditioning (HVAC)	Use slower speed fans Replace hard duct surfaces with ducts covered by a duct liner Install duct silencers Reroute ducts Replace air handler with a quieter version

(Continued)

Table 6.5 (Continued)

Problem	Solution	Examples
Interior Noise Sources	Close gaps between walls and floors with sealant	
	Extend the wall from structural floor to structural ceiling	
	Replace hollow wood doors with solid doors	
	Place doors to avoid spillover	Don't pair up doors next to each other
		Don't place doors directly across the hall from each other
	Locate classrooms away from noise sources	Cafeteria
		Gym
		Woodshop
		Band room
	Construct walls with sound absorption capability	
	Avoid poor classroom set-ups	Open-plan classrooms
		Background noise is not random: another intelligible signal such as another teacher's voice
		Hard ceiling, hard walls, and hard tile floor
		Window/wall-mounted air conditioning units
Exterior Noise	Install tight-fitting seals in walls, doors, and windows	
	Use double-paned glass on windows	
	Locate classrooms away from noise sources	Airplane flyovers
		Busy roads
		Idling school buses
		Playgrounds
		Playing fields
		Exterior mechanical equipment
		Dumpsters being emptied
		Lawn mowers
		Noisy machinery in nearby buildings

SOURCES: Kollie (2006); Nixon (2004); Seep, Glosemeyer, Hulce, Linn, and Aytar (2000).

The next physical aspect that affects understanding in the classroom is *distance*. Sound level (loudness) decreases the farther away the listener is from the source of the sound. Sound pressure decreases by six decibels every time the distance between the source and the listener is doubled. Distance changes the signal-to-noise ratio. For example, if the S/N is +10 when the teacher is five feet away from the student, the S/N is about +4 when the teacher moves across the room to ten feet away. The most effective way to reduce the effect of distance is to move closer to the listener. Teachers often move throughout the classroom repeating instructions to the students, increasing and decreasing the distance between them and the students in different areas of the classroom. Speaking louder is ineffective because it changes the acoustic characteristics of the teacher's voice as well as adding to vocal strain on the teacher. Alternatives are needed to account for the effect of distance.

One way to improve the signal-to-noise ratio and limit the effect of distance is to have the teacher use an *assistive listening device* (ALD). Assistive listening devices allow the teacher to wear a microphone and to transmit a clear sound to the student(s). ALDs have transmitters that use an FM or infrared signal to deliver the sound either to a loudspeaker (or speakers) in the classroom, or directly into the child's personal listening device (hearing aid/cochlear implant). Systems that deliver sound through speaker(s) in the classroom are called *soundfield systems*. Systems that deliver sound directly to individual students are called *personal systems*. Assistive listening devices raise the signal-to-noise ratio, improve speech intelligibility, and reduce vocal strain on the teacher. In order for soundfield systems to be effective, the room must not be reverberant and the amplified sound must not become noise for adjacent classrooms. Assistive listening devices transmit only the teacher's voice unless the children use an auxiliary microphone.

Essential Practice #26

> The *Ling Sound Check* is the quickest, most efficient way to perform ongoing device and hearing monitoring, and it's easy!

DAILY DEVICE MONITORING: YOUR RESPONSIBILITY

Teachers need to monitor listening devices daily in an accurate manner to be sure the devices are working and also to note when a child's perception could be improved by readjusting a device. An efficient and appropriate way to assess a device in the classroom is through the "Ling Sound Check" (see Figure 6.17). An audiologist and teacher of the deaf, Daniel Ling, devised a way to assess the range of speech sounds by presenting these sounds to the child and monitoring the child's responses. Dr. Ling (Ling, 2002) selected each sound because of its unique acoustic properties and/or its potential for confusion with another sound. The sounds are:

The sound -o- as in "hot"

This sound is a high-intensity sound with low-frequency components and should be the most easily perceived by the child. If the child cannot detect this sound, the hearing device requires significant reconfiguration. But first, be sure the device is turned on and the battery isn't dead.

/s/ as in "sin," /sh/ as in "shin," and /th/ as in "thin"

These are high-frequency, low-intensity sounds. If the child confuses these sounds with each other, or does not hear the sound at all, the audiologist can attempt to remedy this by increasing the high-frequency responses of the hearing aid(s) or cochlear implant(s).

The sounds -oo- as in "hoot" and -ee- as in "heat"

These sounds have similar first formants, but different second formants and are often confused with each other. The audiologist will attempt to remediate this by reprogramming the middle frequencies.

The sound /m/ as in "meet"

This sound has acoustical properties similar to -oo- and -ee- and can be confused with those sounds. The audiologist should attempt to boost the low-frequency response of the device to increase the perception of the nasal resonance of the /m/ sound.

Figure 6.17 Checking a Child's Listening

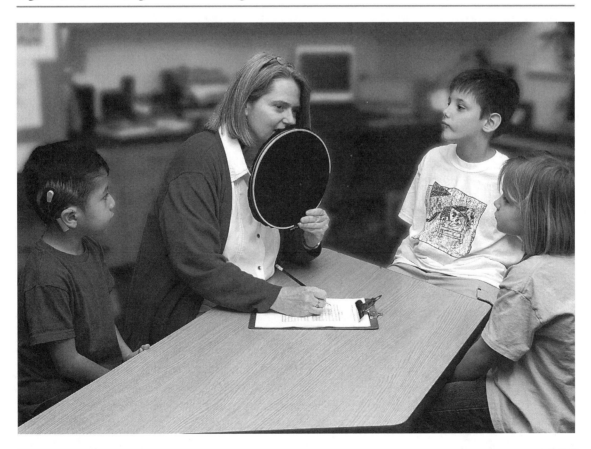

SOURCE: Photographed by John Zimmermann.

HOW TO GIVE THE LING SOUND CHECK

When conducting the Ling Sound Check, use the following guidelines:

- Cover your mouth. This is a listening-only task.

- Begin by developing a detection response to each of the sounds. Say the sound and then have the child indicate in an age-appropriate manner whether or not she has detected the sound. Require at least two confirmations.

- If you have a student with a cochlear implant who cannot detect any of these sounds, contact the implant audiologist. All children with cochlear implants should be able at least to detect all the Ling sounds.

- After the child can detect the sounds, begin to assess discrimination by requiring him to imitate what he heard you say. Again confirm with two attempts. This time, use the *Estes Sound Confusion Matrix* (see Figure 6.18). For example, if you say -oo- and the child says -ee-, place an X in the corresponding box. It is not important that the child's speech matches yours, but that the child indicates awareness by approximating the sound you made and producing different sounds for different stimuli.

- Use a normal voice. You may need to raise the volume of your voice or elongate the sound in the initial stages as a child learns to respond to the task, but as soon as the child has learned the task, present the sound at a normal, conversational level, saying each sound briefly, without emphasis.

- Note your distance from the child. You may need to be close to the child when teaching the task. As the child becomes familiar with the procedure, you should be no closer than three feet away, and begin moving farther and farther from the child with practice. A child with appropriately fitted hearing aid(s) and/or cochlear implant(s) should be able to respond correctly to a sound when it is presented eight feet from his ear.

- Control for background noise. Be aware that performing the Ling Sound Check in a noisy environment could potentially affect the child's responses. Teachers often assess the child's abilities in noise to determine the extent of its effects.

- Know how you expect the child to respond. You may only be asking the child to respond to the sound by indicating that he heard it. You may be asking the child to repeat what you said or in some other way identify what specific sound he heard.

- Whatever your expectation level, it is important that you note whether the child performed as expected. Any change in his response to the sounds is important for you to note and to share with the audiologist. These differences could be indications of problems with the device, or a change in the child's hearing level. Either problem requires appropriate remediation by the audiologist.

- Monitor the rate at which you present the sounds. Do not present the sounds at a predictable rate or rhythm. Insert long pauses before saying the sound. This will require the child to wait for a sound before responding. Predictability encourages guessing. Allow the child to hear silence. Often when the child hears nothing she will guess that you are presenting one of the quiet sounds /s/, /sh/, or /th/. You need to know if the child is guessing at these sounds by presenting silence either through long pauses, or by encouraging the child to say "Nothing" when you don't say a sound.

- Vary the order in which you present the sounds. This removes the extra clue of process of elimination. Presenting each sound more than once will also diminish the clues of elimination and will provide confirmation of the child's responses.
- Be quick about it. Once the child has learned this procedure, it should take no longer than 20 to 30 seconds to complete. Keep records. Keep track of each child's responses so that you can note responses that differ from typical performance. You can also use these records to track the child's progress as his ability matures.

Figure 6.18 Estes Sound Confusion Matrix

Stimulus

Response		o	oo	ee	m	s	sh	∅
	o							
	oo							
	ee							
	m							
	s							
	sh							
	∅							

SUMMARY

This chapter presented 26 essential practices that explain the fundamentals of listening and speaking in the classroom. These practices are:

1. Language is made up of five major systems. A breakdown in any of the systems will influence all the other systems. Children must learn the rules of each system.

2. The semantic system describes meaning at the word, phrase, and sentence level. Words, phrases, and sentences can have more than one meaning, and meanings can be concrete or abstract.

3. The morphology system is composed of root words, prefixes, suffixes, and other parts of speech that change the meaning of words. Children must begin to learn about these rules at a very early age.

4. Syntax refers to the order of words in sentences. Children must hear word order in structured presentations to assimilate order into their growing language.

5. The pragmatics system is another system of language. This system tells us who can say what to whom, when, where, and how. If a child violates these rules, he is often thought of as "odd" or "rude." Pragmatic skills require direct instruction in most instances.

6. The phonology system allows us to describe actual speech as separate from language. Children who are deaf or hard of hearing need incidental and didactic instruction in learning the rules of speech.

7. There is a difference between knowing the labels of the parts of speech (e.g., noun, verb, etc.) and having usable examples of those labels in one's vocabulary (e.g., dog, run). Deaf children usually struggle at the level of word meaning as well as word labels.

8. Provide the child with experience understanding and using the adverbial system, which is an integral component of the ability to apply thinking skills, and which connects higher thought and language. Asking and answering adverbial types of questions is a key to higher-order thinking.

9. Language beyond the early preschool years rapidly becomes very complex and includes challenging constructions that are often beyond the grasp of many young children with hearing loss unless they receive intense listening and language intervention.

10. Language is a very complicated topic to study. The more you learn about how children learn language, the better you will be able to teach them. Learn the rules of language yourself.

11. Human beings like to make sense of the world by making patterns and fitting things together. Language has patterns and is modular. We can

fit our thoughts into the modules of language to communicate very complex ideas.

12. The teacher must account for the biological, environmental, and cognitive factors that affect a child's language development. In addition, the teacher must interact conversationally in relevant ways to account for these factors.

13. The child uses all the clues available to him to understand what is said to him and to incorporate new elements (e.g., words, morphemes, or phrase structure) into his language system. He accesses all that is comprehensible. If a language stimulus is not comprehensible, then he cannot incorporate it into his language system, and it must be specifically taught.

14. Spoken language and thinking go hand in hand. Always work from a base of meaningful activities, focusing on the concept, or thought, as well as on speech and language. Keep the connection between thought and language foremost in your mind as you work with children who are deaf or hard of hearing.

15. The unique physical aspects of the hearing and speech mechanisms in each child affect the approach you will take when helping that child learn to communicate. Each child is different, and you need to individualize your approaches and techniques.

16. There is a direct link between what a child hears and what he says. Understanding the relationship between the acoustic (sound) properties of speech and a child's level of hearing (as shown on an audiogram) will help you target stimulation to the individual child's listening needs. The audiogram will also indicate the type of loss. Consult the child's aided audiogram (i.e., what he hears with his hearing aid and/or cochlear implant) to help determine appropriate instructional objectives and procedures.

17. Teachers need to have an understanding of a child's audiogram and what it means in relation to what the child will be able to hear in the classroom.

18. When helping a child learn to listen to speech, always present sounds that have noticeable differences. This is necessary so the child can learn to discriminate one sound from another. If we don't make sounds noticeably different, the child will merely be guessing.

19. Always teach new speech skills in coarticulation (i.e., vowel and consonant combined) so the child can hear information from the transitions between sounds.

20. Speaking in close range to the child's hearing aids is most important when teaching the lowest and highest frequency sounds.

21. Talk closer to the child's ear. Don't talk louder.

22. Children need to practice hearing and using speech with varied duration.

23. When asking a child to discriminate between two sounds, always make sure that the differences between the sounds are far enough apart for his brain to perceive.

24. Careful, ongoing monitoring of a listening device and the auditory environment improves the chances that a child will make progress in listening and understanding sounds.

25. Children with normal hearing are able to block out background noises; children with hearing losses have difficulty doing this. Be sure to reduce background noise to the maximum extent possible, especially in the classroom, where noise coming through a hearing aid or cochlear implant can easily drown out the teacher's voice.

26. The *Ling Sound Check* is the quickest, most efficient way to perform ongoing device and hearing monitoring, and it's easy!

Resource A

Organizations and Agencies Serving Children With Hearing Losses

Organizations' and Agencies' Web Sites	
Alexander Graham Bell Association for the Deaf	www.agbell.org
American Academy of Audiology	www.audiology.org
American Association of Home-Based Early Interventionists	www.aahbei.org
American Society for Deaf Children	www.asdc.org
American Speech-Language-Hearing Association	www.asha.org
Council for Exceptional Children	www.cec.sped.org
Cued Speech Center	www.cuedspeech.org
Early Hearing Detection and Intervention Program—Centers for Disease Control	www.cdc.gov/ncbddd/ehdi
Gallaudet University—National Information Center on Deafness	www.clerccenter.gallaudet.edu

(Continued)

(Continued)

Organizations' and Agencies' Web Sites	
Hands and Voices	www.handsandvoices.org
National Association of the Deaf	www.nad.org
National Center for Hearing Assessment and Management—Utah State University	www.infanthearing.org
National Institute on Deafness and Other Communication Disorders (NIDCD)	www.nidcd.nih.gov
Network of Educators of Children With Cochlear Implants (NECCI)	www.childrenshearing.org/custom/necci.html
The Center	center.uncg.edu
Oral Deaf Education	www.oraldeafed.org
Assistive Listening Devices	
Audio Enhancement	www.audioenhancement.com
AudioLink Services	www.audiolinks.com
Lightspeed Technologies	www.lightspeed-tek.com
Cochlear Implants	
Advanced Bionics	www.bionicear.com
Cochlear Corporation	www.cochlear.com
Med-El Corporation	www.medel.com
Hearing Aids and/or Listening Devices	
Oticon	www.oticon.com
Phonak	www.phonak.com
Phonic Ear	www.phonicear.ca
Resound	www.gnresound.com
Siemens	www.siemens-hearing.com
Sonic Innovations	www.sonici.com
Sonovation	www.avrsono.com
Widex	www.widex.com

Resource B
Assessments

Language	
Assessment Tool	*Age or Grade Range*
Boehm Test of Basic Concepts—3rd Edition (Boehm-3)	Kindergarten to Grade 2
Boehm Test of Basic Concepts–Preschool—3rd Edition (Boehm P-3)	3 yrs., 0 mos. to 5 yrs., 11 mos.
Clinical Evaluation of Language Function—4th Edition (CELF-4)	5 yrs., 0 mos. to 21 yrs., 11 mos.
Clinical Evaluation of Language Function—Preschool—2nd Edition (CELF-P2)	3 yrs., 0 mos. to 6 yrs., 11 mos.
Comprehensive Assessment of Spoken Language (CASL)	3 yrs., 0 mos. to 21 yrs., 11 mos.
Expressive One-Word Picture Vocabulary Test (EOWPVT)	2 yrs., 6 mos. to 18 yrs., 11 mos.
Expressive Vocabulary Test (EVT)	2 yrs., 6 mos. to 90+ yrs.
Grammatical Analysis of Elicited Language—Pre-Sentence (GAEL-P)	3 yrs., 0 mos. to 6 yrs., 11 mos.
MacArthur-Bates Communicative Development Inventories (CDIs)	8 mos. to 30 mos.
OWLS Listening Comprehension and Oral Expression Scale (OWLS LC/OE)	3 yrs., 0 mos. to 21 yrs., 11 mos.
OWLS Written Expression Scale (OWLS WE)	5 yrs., 0 mos. to 21 yrs., 11 mos.
Peabody Picture Vocabulary Test—4th Edition (PPVT-4)	2 yrs., 6 mos. to 90+ yrs.
Preschool Language Assessment Instrument—2nd Edition (PLAI-2)	3 yrs., 0 mos. to 5 yrs., 11 mos.
Preschool Language Scale—4th Edition (PLS-4)	birth to 6 yrs., 11 mos.
Receptive One Word Picture Vocabulary Test (ROWPVT)	2 yrs., 0 mos. to 18 yrs., 11 mos.
SKI*HI Language Development Scale (LDS)	birth to 5 yrs.

(Continued)

(Continued)

Language	
Assessment Tool	*Age or Grade Range*
Structured Photographic Elicited Language Test (SPELT)	4 yrs., 0 mos. to 9 yrs., 11 mos.
Test for Auditory Comprehension of Language—3rd Edition (TACL-3)	3 yrs., 0 mos. to 9 yrs., 11 mos.
Test of Language Development—Primary—3rd Edition (TOLD-P3)	4 yrs., 0 mos. to 8 yrs., 11 mos.
Development/Intelligence	
Assessment Tool	*Age Range*
Assessment, Evaluation and Programming (AEPS)	birth to 36 mos.
Battelle Developmental Inventory—2nd Edition	birth to 7 yrs., 11 mos.
Bayley Scales of Infant Development—2nd Edition	1 mo. to 30 mos.
Bracken Basic Concept Scale–Revised	3 yrs., 0 mos. to 6 yrs., 11 mos.
Brigance Inventory of Early Development 2nd Edition (IED-II)	birth to 7 yrs., 11 mos.
Central Institute for the Deaf—Preschool Performance Scale (PPS)	2 yrs., 0 mos. to 5 yrs., 5 mos.
Comprehensive Test of Nonverbal Intelligence (CTONI)	6 yrs., 0 mos. to 18 yrs., 11 mos.
Developmental Programming for Infants & Young Children Volume 2 (DPIYC-2)	birth to 36 mos.
Hawaii Early Learning Profile–HELP	birth to 3 yrs., 6 mos.
Learning Accomplishment Profile 3rd Edition (LAP-3)	36 mos. to 72 mos.
Leiter International Performance Scale–Revised (Leiter-R)	2 yrs., 0 mos. to 20 yrs., 11 mos.
Portage Guide Birth to Six	birth to 5 yrs., 11 mos.
Progressive Matrices (Raven)	5 yrs., 0 mos. to 11 yrs., 11 mos.
Rosetti Infant Toddler Scale	birth to 36 mos.
Universal Nonverbal Intelligence Test (UNIT)	5 yrs., 0 mos. to 17 yrs., 11 mos.
Vineland Adaptive Behavior Scales—2nd Edition	birth to 90+ yrs.
Weschler Intelligence Scale for Children—4th Edition (WISC-IV)	6 yrs., 0 mos. to 16 yrs., 11 mos.
Weschler Preschool and Primary Scales of Intelligence—3rd Edition (WPPSI-III)	2 yrs., 6 mos. to 7 yrs., 3 mos.
Woodcock-Johnson Tests of Cognitive Ability—3rd Edition (WJ-III)	2 yrs., 0 mos. to 99 yrs., 11 mos.

Achievement/Reading	
Assessment Tool	*Age or Grade Range*
Comprehensive Test of Phonological Processing (CTOPP)	5 yrs., 0 mos. to 24 yrs., 11 mos.
Diagnostic Achievement Battery—3rd Edition (DAB-3)	6 yrs., 0 mos. to 14 yrs., 11 mos.
Gray Oral Reading Test—4th Edition (GORT-4)	6 yrs., 0 mos. to 18 yrs., 11 mos.
Informal Reading Inventory—6th Edition	Preprimer to Grade 12
Johns Basic Reading Inventory—9th Edition	Preprimer to Grade 12
Key Math—Revised	Kindergarten to Grade 9
Peabody Individual Achievement Test—Revised (PIAT-R)	5 yrs., 0 mos. to 8 yrs., 11 mos.
Pre-Reading Inventory of Phonological Awareness (PIPA)	4 yrs., 0 mos. to 6 yrs., 11 mos.
Stanford Achievement Test—10th Edition and Otis-Lennon School Ability Test—8th Edition (OLSAT 8)	Kindergarten to Grade 12
Test of Early Math Ability—3rd Edition (TEMA-3)	4 yrs., 0 mos. to 8 yrs., 11 mos.
Test of Early Reading Ability—3rd Edition (TERA-3)	3 yrs., 6 mos. to 8 yrs., 6 mos.
Test of Early Written Language—2nd Edition (TEWL-2)	3 yrs., 0 mos. to 10 yrs., 11 mos.
Test of Reading Comprehension—3rd Edition (TORC-3)	7 yrs., 0 mos. to 17 yrs., 11 mos.
Test of Written Language—3rd Edition (TWL-3)	7 yrs., 6 mos. to 17 yrs., 11 mos.
Weschler Individual Achievement Test—2nd Edition (WIAT-II)	4 yrs., 6 mos. to 85 yrs.
Woodcock-Johnson Tests of Achievement—3rd Edition (WJ-III)	2 yrs., 0 mos. to 99 yrs., 11 mos.
Woodcock Reading Mastery Test—Revised (WRMT-R)	5 yrs., 0 mos. to 75+ yrs.
Speech Production	
Assessment Tool	*Age Range*
Arizona Articulation Proficiency Scale–3rd Edition (AAPS-3)	1 yr., 6 mos. to 18 yrs., 11 mos.
Central Institute for the Deaf Phonetic Inventory	NA
Goldman-Fristoe Test of Articulation–2nd Edition	2 yrs., 0 mos. to 11 yrs.
Identifying Early Phonological Needs in Children with Hearing Loss (IEPN)	NA
Ling Phonetic—Phonologic Speech Evaluation	NA

(Continued)

(Continued)

Speech Perception/Intelligibility (no age or grade ranges)

Word Recognition—Open Set:
       Phonetically Balanced Kindergarten lists (PBK-50)
       Glendonald Assessment of Speech Perception (GASP Words)

Word Recognition—Closed Set:
       Northwestern University—Children's Perception of Speech (NU-CHIPS)
       Auditory Numbers Test (ANT)
       Word Intelligibility by Picture Identification (WIPI)
       Central Institute for the Deaf spondee Words (CID W-1)
       Central Institute for the Deaf CV, VC, and CVC Words (CID W-22)

Word Recognition—Closed Set and Open Set: Early Speech Perception Test (ESP & ESP Low Verbal)

Sentences—Open Set:
       Central Institute for the Deaf Sentences (CID Sentences)
       Glendonald Assessment of Speech Perception (GASP Questions)

Resource C

Sound-Object Associations

Ellen A. Rhoades, EdS
Certified Auditory Verbal Therapist
www.auditoryverbaltraining.com

Long before babies speak words or know their meanings, they hear sounds and remember them (Jusczyk, 1997). This involves associating a sound with a *referent,* a meaningful object or action. Parents of babies with normal hearing consistently associate sounds to items or actions (Harding, 1983; Norris & Hoffman, 1994). Young babies become familiar with frequently heard sounds before they understand and say words. *Sound-object association* activities can facilitate listening for children with hearing losses,

Formerly referred to as "learning to listen" sounds, *sound-object associations* are used with children who are deaf or hard of hearing engaging in auditory learning. Linking a sound to a meaningful referent is an important activity for auditory intervention Some goals that are addressed through facilitating the development of sound-object associations are:

- To encourage the child to attend to sounds

- To facilitate the recognition that sounds are different

- To help the child understand that different sounds have different meaning

- To develop auditory imprints (also known as auditory schema or stored perceptual representations) for specific sounds or language-based phonemes

- To highlight critical parameters used in spoken language

- To engage the child in turn-taking and joint attention behavioral interactions

- To stimulate fluent movement of the child's articulators needed for speech

- To help the child experiment with producing different sounds

- To integrate and synchronize physical and social behaviors into vocal interactions

- To develop "communicative intention"

- To develop auditory familiarity with the spoken language

- To enable the child to participate in communicative interactions before he or she understands the concept of communicating

Young children need to be actively engaged in the learning and listening process. Parents should therefore use toys and common actions, as opposed to pictures, during sound-object association activities. Sound-object activities are meant to be meaningful as well as actively enjoyable for both adult and child—not passive, rote drill work (Stark, Ansel, & Bond, 1988). Each time children hear a sound in a different context, it restructures the auditory schema of a particular sound (Norris & Hoffman, 1994). For this reason, we should vary how we use each sound.

Start with just one, two, or three sound-object associations when first implementing sound-object activities and introduce more associations after a few exposures. Young infants categorize their newly learned concepts (Hasegawa & Miyashita, 2002), so follow this natural pattern and present sound-object associations categorically for ease in planning and learning. For example, avoid mixing transportation vehicle sounds with animal sounds in the same session at first. Use toys that are easily recognizable and have simple, obvious representations. For example, "moo" obviously represents a toy cow. Choose toy animals in standing rather than sitting positions. Choose generic rather than fanciful representations of objects. For example, use typical vehicles such as a sedan rather than a convertible. However, if all you have available is a convertible, then by all means use that. Children 18 months and older may be able to work with toys that are less representational; that is, toys where dimensions or colors are less realistic. Avoid toys that produce a sound while being moved, because these sounds typically take precedence over speech. If the toy is battery-operated, remove the battery during the session. As the child gains success, vary the objects you use for each sound, that is, use a variety of cars to expand the child's concept of what that associated sound represents. Multiple objects used as the same referent also serve to maintain the child's interest.

Provide a variety of table-top props with which the objects interact. Examples of table-top props are a plastic fence, a gas station or airport hangar, a train track, a barn, an oval piece of blue paper representing a small water pond, some small pebbles, and twigs retrieved from outdoors. The props lend themselves to more interesting activities, provide greater opportunities for repeated vocalization of sounds, and add to the variety of connected language that accompanies the sounds being made. Young infants seem to attend more to visual objects when they have an auditory stimulus associated with them.

Give special attention to voiceless sounds, plosives, fricatives, and affricates. These are phonemes that are whispered, not voiced (e.g., /h/, /t/, /p/, /k/, /s/, /f/, /ch/, and /sh/). These high-frequency, low-intensity sounds are often difficult for children to hear when couched within whole words, since the louder vowels in the word supersede the whispered phonemes. It is therefore important that these voiceless sounds be used without vowels during sound-object association activities. Table C.1 provides examples of sound-object associations that are based on my experiences as someone with a hearing loss and as an Auditory-Verbal Master Clinician for more than 30 years.

Pointers to Remember

1. Assess current associations. Determine if the child is already making sound-object associations and use the "association" the child has naturally made. For example, a child may already associate "toot toot" with a train moving. If you were planning on using the train for the "chchchch" sound, engage in a train playing activity where the "chchchch" sound is made only when the train is starting up and the "toot toot" sound is made when the train moves, or use another referent for the "chchchch" sound.

2. Check comprehension. From time to time, check on the child's understanding of the sound-object associations you are making. While it is unrealistic to ask babies to make appropriate selections, toddlers one year and older are capable of choosing the requested target object (Woodward & Hoyne, 1999). For example, after playing with a garage, some cars, a fire truck, some airplanes, and a paper landing strip, ask the child for a vehicle by sound while holding out a hand or receptacle and wait for the appropriate response. Comprehension checks should be done naturally, meaningfully, and in a playful manner. Keep a record of those sounds that the child understands without the use of visual cues.

3. An effective auditory-verbal strategy that should be used with sound-object association activities is that "hearing always comes first." The adult should vocalize the sound before showing the child the item.

4. Develop voice-action synchrony. Change the pitch, duration, rate, loudness, and so forth of your voice as you change the movements of the object. For example, as you move the toy rabbit up and down, say, "Hop" each time you pick the rabbit up.

5. Know when to move on. Typically, when the child understands most of the sounds, it's time to move on to using the words and dropping the sounds; that is, "chchchch" becomes "train."

6. Expect inconsistency. Young children do not always perform in a consistent manner. The 80 percent target of many school objectives may be unrealistic for young children. As long as the child demonstrates that he clearly understands that a particular sound is associated with the referent, then comprehension for a handful of animal sounds and another handful of vehicle sounds is all that is needed. At this point, the young child has demonstrated understanding that sounds are meaningful and differentiated, and that exposure to varied auditory schema has occurred.

7. Be creative. Daily activities should be presented in a variety of ways. Incorporating seasonal themes facilitates creativity and develops meaningful associations. For example, ghosts say "Oooooo" on Halloween; we click our tongues when playing with cowboy toys; Santa Claus says "Ho ho ho!" at Christmas; "Mmmmm" is what we say when eating Halloween or Valentine's Day candy; "Hop hop hop" is what the Easter bunny does; "Sssss" is what we say as we fill up the inflatable wading pool with water.

8. Use multiple toys in multiple contexts to avoid boredom and facilitate flexibility. Vary the playful situation each day. One day, small boats can slosh around in a large plastic bowl halfway filled with water. The next day, those same boats can imaginatively "sail" across a blue piece of paper. The following day, little plastic people or animals can board a larger toy boat. Moreover, use appropriate sounds when reading children's books. The hardest part of the adult's job is to be creative because children can become bored with repetition.

9. Separate special toys. Because therapy materials involve adult participation, parents should be advised to keep these toys separate from the child's regular toys. Young children come to view these toys as being special, and that provides even more of an incentive for them to engage in play therapy with their parents.

10. Make interactions enjoyable. Caution parents that these activities should be fun without applying pressure on the child to talk. After all, the child is just learning to listen. With sufficient exposure over time and across multiple situations, the child will begin to vocalize. Talking should be a comfortable, spontaneous act that occurs subsequent to multiple sound exposures (Meltzoff, 1999).

11. Transition from sounds to words as soon as possible. When the child can identify many of the objects based on the associated sounds made by the adult, transition to making word-object associations by naming the animals and vehicles. Some children may have difficulty making this transition to a higher symbolic level due to an excessive amount of time spent on sounds. Difficulty with transitioning from sound-object to word-object associations may also be indicative of co-occurring developmental disorders such as autism spectrum disorder or learning disabilities such as auditory processing disorder.

12. Follow the developmental sequence of acquisition. These are:
    Step 1: Child will identify the object by the sound
    Step 2: Child *may* vocalize the sound, either by imitation or spontaneously
    Step 3: Child will identify the object by its name and sound
    Step 4: Child will identify the object by its name
    Step 5: Child *may* vocalize the name, either by imitation or spontaneously

The sounds presented in the following table are sufficient for exposing children to many features of speech, particularly those of duration, intensity, pitch, voicing and nonvoicing, as well as some basic consonants and vowels. Adults need not incorporate additional sounds into play therapy because too many may inhibit progress toward lexical learning.

Sound	Toy	Characteristics	Suggestions
			Transportation Vehicles
Aaaaaah	Airplane	Stimulates use of strong low-frequency vowel. Generally easy for all children, no matter the degree of loss.	Use among the first sounds. Exaggerate suprasegmental features (inflection and duration). Fly plane up and down to mimic vocal duration. Listen for suprasegmental variations if the child spontaneously imitates the sound. If child uses a monotone voice, sing the sound, exaggerating intonation and incorporating rhythmic, whole body movements.
Buhbuhbuhbuh	Bus	Stimulates use of lip articulators. One of the first consonants babies with normal hearing produce.	Sing the sound using various rhythms to synchronize with bus movements. Since /b/ and /m/ look the same, do not let child see lips while adult says the sound. Vocalize the sound only when moving the bus. To highlight intensity differences, use small bus for soft sounds and large bus for loud sounds.
Oooooooo	Fire truck, ambulance, or police car	Stimulates use of intonation or pitch variations. A favorite of children.	Vocalize from high to low and low to high while imitating the sound of a siren. Gradually expand duration. If a parent is not able to vary pitch on this sound, choose "eeeee." Synchronize sound with truck movement in both voicing and pitch. If a fire truck is not available, use ambulance or police car. Focus on intonation without visual cues.
Brrrrrrrr	Car	Stimulates use of lip articulators. Also known as "blowing raspberries."	Parents may be more comfortable practicing this first at home. Synchronize lip-trilling sound with car movements in both length and rhythm. Accept any lip or tongue trilling efforts from child.
Ptptptptpt	Boat	Some therapists prefer using the "p-p-p" sound. Develops familiarity with high-frequency sounds.	Sound should be produced with a whisper, so help parents practice saying it until there is complete absence of a vowel. Explain the logic behind this to parents: vowels "drown out" high-frequency consonants; we want acoustic clarity when imprinting consonants on the child's brain. Strive for voice-action synchrony. Presence and absence of sound associates with presence and absence of movement; rhythm of voice associates with movement of boat.

(Continued)

Sound	Toy	Characteristics	Suggestions
Chchchchch	Train	Stimulates high-frequency consonants, pushing tongue to roof of mouth, and for possible later use when comparing short sounds with longer sounds such as "ch" as compared to "sh."	Avoid saying "choo-choo-choo." Whispering highlights the consonant as described above. Check parents' ability to produce without the vowel. Try to find a train that does not make a sound as turning on the sound will be too tempting for the child and the objective will not be reached. Fun noises compete unfavorably with human speech. If a noiseless train is unavailable, remove batteries. Allow child to play with another train that makes noises; save the noiseless one for therapy.
Animals			
Mooooooo	Cow	Stimulates use of strong, basic vowel.	Use a low voice, dropping it to bass. Children find this change interesting. Do not vary pitch or loudness, but do vary duration. Synchronize your voice with how the cow is moved.
Repeated tongue clicking	Horse	Stimulates use of tongue articulator.	The child may want to see your mouth when you make this sound, so try to produce it without visible movement of your articulators. Child may not be able to produce this, but objective is for child to notice it as being different from other sounds. Synchronize the rhythm and speed of your clicks with the speed and rhythm of a trotting or galloping horse.
Meeow	Cat	Facilitates two-syllable vowel transitions.	Make an effort to sound like a cat. Be sure the "ow" part is nicely rounded. Play with cows and cats in one activity so that the child becomes familiar with hearing the differences between "moo" and "meeow."
Woof-woof, arf-arf, or ruff-ruff	Dog	Introduces voiceless, high-frequency sound in final position.	Do not use "bow-wow" as the /b/ is already used for bus and the "ow" is already used for cat; each sound should be uniquely associated with each toy. Say this sound softly (not loud), so that the fricative /f/ will be heard, especially if said within close proximity to the child's ear. Make the sound rise from your chest as if you were barking.

Sound	Toy	Characteristics	Suggestions
Ssssssss	Snake	Facilitates whispering and use of voiceless consonant. Also checks whether child's hearing prosthesis is working.	Typically, children younger than two years of age will not produce this sound. Babies and toddlers love to have adults whisper in their ear. Children with aided hearing thresholds worse than 35 dB may have difficulty hearing this sound. Be sure you are in close proximity to the child's ear. If child is fearful of snakes, use this sound to represent the use of a hose to water flowers, to put out a pretend fire, or to put gas in a toy car.
Quack quack	Duck	Highlights the fricative /k/ in initial and final positions.	Use a low voice (bass). Good for working on duration changes; make both long and short quacks to mimic the toy duck's actions. If child does not respond to the sound, you may need to move closer to his ear and highlight the /k/ sound more specifically.
Hop hop hop	Rabbit	Highlights action-oriented word and fricatives /h/ and /p/. Develops awareness of voicing and nonvoicing contrasts.	Use the sound in a whisper and voiced. Dim lights and whisper what a toy rabbit is doing. Turn on the light when you voice the movement of the rabbit. Whispering helps child to hear the high-frequency sounds; changing the lighting helps to highlight the concept of voicing and nonvoicing.
Oink oink	Pig	Highlights the first diphthong and the "nk" final sound.	Follow rules of voice-action synchrony. Sing "Old McDonald had a farm" and read children's stories about farm animals that include pigs.
Ba-a-a-a-a	Sheep	Develops awareness of variation with fundamental vowel.	Provides for a listening contrast between "aaaah" and "a-a-a-a." The difference is more noticeable as vowels are prolonged in duration. This is an appropriate time to play with both animal (sheep) and vehicle (airplane), such as having a little sheep ride in a big toy airplane.
Squeak (or) Eeek	Mouse	Develops awareness of falsetto voice.	In a very high-pitched voice, adult uses either sound to represent mouse. Follow rules of voice-action synchrony. Say the squeaking sound as a wind-up mouse moves around on the floor or table.

(Continued)

(Continued)

Sound	Toy	Characteristics	Suggestions
Whistling like a bird	Bird	Facilitates use of mouth articulator.	Most young children will not be able to whistle, but many will spontaneously try by vocalizing a falsetto "oooo" or "eeeee." Try to imitate loud bird sounds that are heard outside in an otherwise quiet environment.
Actions			
Mmmmm	To indicate food's tastiness	Facilitates eventual production of sound in isolation.	Pretend to eat foods, saying "Mmmm, it's good." with naturally occurring inflection (rise and fall in pitch). Avoid overuse of this sound; dropping it after child hears and produces it without saying "mba."
Shhhhh	To indicate the need for quiet	Facilitates eventual production of sound in isolation.	Pretend a doll is sleeping; turn off lights and tip-toe with a finger over your mouth saying "Shhh."
Smacking lips	To indicate sucking or kissing	Stimulates use of pursed lips as articulators.	Use as the drinking sound when feeding doll a bottle. Let cows and horses move to water trough on toy farm and lap make-believe water. As usual, engage in voice-action synchrony.
T-t-t-t	To indicate the ticking of a clock	Facilitates eventual production of the voiceless sound.	You can use a finger moving back and forth to represent the rhythmic movement of a clock's second hand. The child should hear a loud clock ticking when in close proximity. Do not insert a vowel sound. Hide a clock that makes a loud ticking sound and search for it.
K-k-k-k G-g-g-g	To indicate coughing, gargling	Stimulates back tongue articulators. Facilitates eventual production of voiced and voiceless consonant equivalents.	Take care not to insert a vowel sound with "k-k-k-k." Pretend a baby doll is coughing and gently pat it on its back. Pretend a doll is gargling after brushing its teeth. Have the child watch while you hold water in your mouth, making bubbles with your head tilted back.

Resource D

Commercially Available Curriculum Guides and Materials

MULTICATEGORICAL (LISTENING, LANGUAGE, AND SPEECH)

AuSpLan: Auditory Speech and Language Development

Cottage Acquisition Scales for Listening, Language and Speech (CASLLS)

Listen, Learn and Talk

LISTENING

Functional Auditory Performance Indicators (FAPI)

Listen Up

Speech Perception Instructional Curriculum and Evaluation (SPICE)

Word Associations for Syllable Perception (WASP)

LANGUAGE

Structured Methods in Language Education (SMILE)

Teacher Assessment of Grammatical Structures (TAGS)

Teacher Assessment of Spoken Language (TASL)

SPEECH

Ling Phonetic-Phonologic Speech Evaluation

Step by Step: The Foundations of Intelligible Speech

Talk It Up

READING

Benchmark Word Identification Program

Children's Early Intervention for Speech, Language, and Reading (CEI)

Edmark Reading Program

Great Leaps

Jolly Phonics

Lindamood Phoneme Sequencing Program for Reading, Spelling, and Speech (LiPS)

Phonological Awareness Skills Program (PASP)

Reading Recovery

Spatial Awareness Skills Program (SASP)

Specialized Program Individualizing Reading Excellence (S.P.I.R.E)

Sunform Alphabet System

Sing, Spell, Read & Write

Wilson—Fundations

Wilson Reading System

References

About, Inc. (n.d.) *Definition of generalized Wiener process.* Retrieved April 17, 2006, from http://www.economics.about.com/library/glossary/bldef-generalized-wiener-process.htm

Alegria, J., & Lechat, J. (2005). Phonological processing in deaf children: When lipreading and cues are incongruent. *Journal of Deaf Studies and Deaf Education, 10*(2), 122–133.

Anderson, R. C., Wilson, P. T., & Fielding, L. G. (1988). Growth in reading and how children spend their time outside of school. *Reading Research Quarterly, 23*(3), 285–303.

Arehart, K. H., & Yoshinaga-Itano, C. (1999). The role of educators of the deaf in the early identification of hearing loss. *American Annals of the Deaf, 144*(1), 19–23.

Arehart, K. H., Yoshinaga-Itano, C., Thomson, V., Gabbard, S. A., & Brown, A. S. (1998). State of the states: The status of universal newborn hearing screening, assessment, and intervention systems in 16 states. *American Journal of Audiology, 7*(2), 101–114.

Barker, S. E., Lesperance, M. M., & Kileny, P. (2000). Outcome of newborn hearing screening by ABR compared with four different DPOAE pass criteria. *American Journal of Audiology, 9*, 142–148.

Berg, R., & Stork, D. G. (1995). *The physics of sound* (2nd ed.). Englewood Cliffs, NJ: Prentice Hall.

Best, C. T. (1994). The emergence of native-language phonological influences in infants: A perceptual assimilation model. In J. V. Goodman & H. C. Nusbaum (Eds.), *The development of speech perception: The transition from speech sounds to spoken words* (pp. 167–224). Cambridge, MA: MIT.

Biedenstein, J., Davidson, L., & Moog, J. (1995). *SPICE: Speech perception instructional curriculum and evaluation.* St. Louis: Central Institute for the Deaf.

Biever, C. (2004, August 19). Language may shape thought. *NewScientist.com News Service.* Retrieved April 17, 2006, from www.newscientist.com/article.ns?id=dn6303

Bloom, L. (1970). *Language development: Form and function in emerging grammars.* Cambridge, MA: MIT Press.

Boone, D. R., & Plante, E. (1993). *Human communication and its disorders* (2nd ed). Englewood Cliffs, NJ: Prentice Hall.

Brown, R. (1973). *A first language: The early stages.* Cambridge, MA: Harvard University Press.

Bruner, J. S. (1975). The ontogenesis of speech acts. *Journal of Child Language, 2*, 1–40.

Calderon, R. (2000). Parents' involvement in deaf children's education programs as a predictor of child's language, early reading, and social-emotional development. *Journal of Deaf Studies and Deaf Education, 5*, 140–155.

Calderon, R., & Naidu, S. (1999). Further support for the benefits of early identification and intervention for children with hearing loss. *Volta Review, 100*(5), 53–84.

Calvert, D. R., & Silverman, S. R. (1975). *Speech and deafness.* Washington, DC: A. G. Bell Association for the Deaf and Hard of Hearing.

Carnine, D. W., Kameenui, E.J., Silbert, J., & Tarver, S. (2003). *Direct instruction reading* (4th ed.). New York: Prentice-Hall.

Caselli, M. C. (1990). Communicative gestures and first words. In V. Volterra & C. J. Erting (Eds.), *From gesture to language in hearing and deaf children.* Washington, DC: Gallaudet University Press.

CDI Advisory Committee (2003). *MacArthur-Bates Communicative Development Inventories.* Baltimore: Brookes.

Cheng, A. K., Grant, G. D., & Niparko, J. K. (1999). Meta-analysis of pediatric cochlear implant literature. *Annals of Otology, Rhinology and Laryngology, 108,* 124–128.

Clark, M. D. (1991). When the same is different: A comparison of the information processing strategies of deaf and hearing people. *American Annals of the Deaf, 136*(4), 349–359.

Clarke School for the Deaf/Center for Oral Education. (1995). *Speech development and improvement: Clarke curriculum series.* Northampton, MA: Author.

Condon, W. (1976). An analysis of behavioral organization. In W. Stokoe & H. R. Bernard (Eds.), *Sign language studies.* Silver Spring, MD: Linstok Press.

De Boysson-Bardie, B. (1989). A crosslinguistic investigation of vowel formants in babbling. *Journal of Child Language, 16*(1), 1–17.

Denes, P. & Pinson, E. (1993). *The speech chain: The physics and biology of spoken language* (2nd ed.). New York: W. H. Freeman.

Desjardin, J. L., Eisenberg, L. S., & Hodapp, R. M. (2006). Sound beginnings: Supporting families of young deaf children with cochlear implants. *Infants & Young Children, 19*(3), 179–189.

Dickson, S. V., Chard, D. J., & Simmons, D. C. (1993). An integrated reading/writing curriculum: A focus on scaffolding. *LD Forum, 18*(4), 12–16.

Dobrich, W., & Scarborough, H. S. (1984). Form and function in early communication: Language and pointing gestures. *Journal of Experimental Child Psychology, 38*(3), 475–490.

Dolch, E. W. (1948). *Problems in reading.* Champaign, IL: The Garrard Press.

Dunst, C. J., Bruder, M. B. (2002). Valued outcomes of service coordination, early intervention, and natural environments. *Exceptional Children, 68*(3), 361–375.

Easterbrooks, S. R., & Baker, S. (2002). *Language learning in children who are deaf and hard of hearing: Multiple pathways.* Boston: Allyn & Bacon.

Easterbrooks, S. R., & Baker-Hawkins, S. (1995). *Deaf and hard of hearing students: Education Services Guidelines.* Washington, DC: National Association of State Directors of Special Education.

Eliot, L. (1999). *What's going on in there? How the brain and mind develop in the first five years of life.* New York: Random House.

Erber, N. P. (1982). *Auditory training.* Washington, DC: A. G. Bell Association for the Deaf and Hard of Hearing.

Erber, N., & Greer, C. W. (1973). Communication strategies used by teachers at an oral school for the deaf. *Volta Review, 75*(8), 480–485.

Erenberg, S. (1999). Automated auditory brainstem response testing for universal newborn hearing screening. *Otolaryngologic Clinics of North America, 32*(6), 999–1007.

Ertmer, D. J., Leonard, J. S., & Pachuilo, M. P. (2002). Communication intervention for children with cochlear implants: Two case studies. *Language, Speech, and Hearing Services in the Schools, 33*, 206–218.

Estabrooks, W. (1994). *Auditory-verbal therapy for parents and professionals.* Washington, DC: The Alexander Graham Bell Association for the Deaf, Inc.

Estabrooks, W. (Ed.). (2001). *Fifty frequently asked questions about auditory-verbal therapy.* Toronto: Learning to Listen Foundation.

Fair, D. (1998). Motherese. *British Medical Journal, 316*(7133), 753–754.

Ferguson, C. A. (1968). Historical background of universals research. In J. Greenberg, C. Ferguson, & E. Moravcsik (Eds.), *Universals of human languages* (pp. 7–31). Stanford, CA: Stanford University Press.

Feuerstein, R. (1980). *Instrumental enrichment.* Baltimore, MD: University Park Press.

First Words Speech Therapy (2004). *Milestones related to speech therapy.* Retrieved April 17, 2006, from www.fwspeech.com/milestones.php

Flege, J. E. (1995). Second language speech learning: Theory, findings, and problems. In W. Strange (Ed.), *Speech perception and linguistic experience: Issues in cross-language research* (pp. 233–273). Baltimore: York.

Fountas, G. S., & Pinnell, I. C. (1996). *Guided reading: Good first teaching for all children.* Portsmouth, NH: Heinemann.

Fry, D. B. (1999). *The physics of speech.* New York: Cambridge University Press.

Gallagher, P. A., Easterbrooks, S. R., & Malone, D. G. (2006). Universal newborn hearing screening and intervention: Assessing the current collaborative environment in service provision to infants with hearing loss. *Infants and Young Children, 19*(1), 59–71.

Geers, A. E., & Moog, J. S. (1987). Predicting spoken language acquisition of profoundly hearing impaired children. *Journal of Speech and Hearing Disorders, 5*, 84–94.

Geers, A. (1994). Techniques for assessing auditory speech perception and lipreading enhancement in young deaf children. *Volta Review, 96*(5), 85–96.

Gibbons, P. (2002). *Scaffolding language, scaffolding learning.* Portsmouth, NH: Heinemann.

Goldberg, J. (2005). The quivering bundles that let us hear. *Seeing, Hearing and Smelling the World: A Report from the Howard Hughes Medical Institute.* Chevy Chase, MD.

Grimshaw, G., Adelstein, A., Bryden, M. P., & MacKinnon, G. E. (1998). First-language acquisition in adolescence: Evidence for a critical period for verbal language development. *Brain and Learning, 63*, 237–255.

Harding, C. G. (1983). Setting the stage for language acquisition: Communication development in the first year. In R. M. Golinkoff (Ed.), *The transition from prelinguistic to linguistic communication* (pp. 93–113). Hillside, NJ: Erlbaum.

Harris, T. L., & Hodges, R. E. (1995). *The literacy dictionary: The vocabulary of reading and writing.* Newark, DE: International Reading Association.

Harrison, M., Roush, J., & Wallace, J. (2003). Trends in age of identification and intervention in infants with hearing loss. *Ear and Hearing, 24*(1), 89–95.

Hart, B. and Risley, T. (1995). *Meaningful differences in everyday parenting and intellectual development in young American children.* Baltimore: Brookes.

Hasegawa, I. & Miyashita, Y. (2002). Categorizing the world: Expert neurons look into key features. *Nature Neuroscience, 5*(2), 90–91.

Haskins, H. (1949). *A phonetically balanced test of speech discrimination for children.* Unpublished master's thesis, Northwestern University, Evanston, IL.

Honig, B., Diamond, L., & Gutlohn, L. (2000). *Teaching reading sourcebook for kindergarten through eight grade.* Novato, CA: Arena Press.

Hughes, C. (1999, February 19–20). *Auditory management of the child with hearing loss* [workshop]. Atlanta.

Individuals with Disabilities Education Improvement Act—IDEA. (2004). Retrieved April 17, 2006, from www.ed.gov/policy/speced/guid/idea/idea2004.html

Joint Committee on Infant Hearing. (2000). Year 2000 position statement: Principles and guidelines for early hearing detection and intervention programs. *American Journal of Audiology, 9*, 9–29.

Jusczyk, P. (1997). *The discovery of spoken language.* Cambridge: MIT Press.

Jusczyk, P. W., Friederici, A. P., Wessels, J. M., Svenderud, V. Y., & Jusczyk, A. M. (1993). Infants' sensitivity to the sound patterns of native language words. *Journal of Memory and Language, 32*(3), 402–420.

Kelly, L. (1993). Recall of English function words and inflections by skilled and average deaf readers. *American Annals of the Deaf, 138*, 288–296.

Kelly, R. R., Lang, H. G., & Pagliaro, C. M. (2003). Mathematics word problem solving for deaf students: A survey of practices in grades 6–12. *Journal of Deaf Studies and Deaf Education, 8*(2), 104–119.

Kluwin, T. N., Stinson, M. S., & Colarossi, G. M. (2002). Social processes and outcomes of in-school contact between deaf and hearing peers. *Journal of Deaf Studies and Deaf Education, 7*(3), 200–213.

Kollie, E. (2006). Acoustics take the lead in classroom design. *School Planning & Management, 45*(2), 36–40.

Koopmans-van Beinum, F. J., Clement, C. J., & van den Dikkenberg-Pot, I. (2001). Babbling and the lack of auditory speech perception: A matter of coordination? *Developmental Science, 4*(1), 61–70.

Kozulin, A., & Rand, Y. (Eds.). (2002). *Experience of mediated learning: An impact of Feuerstein's theory in education and psychology.* Oxford, UK: Elsevier Science Ltd.

Kuhl, P. K. (2000). Language, mind, and brain: Experience alters perception. In M. S. Gazzaniga (Ed.), *The new cognitive neurosciences* (2nd ed., pp. 99–115). Cambridge, MA: MIT Press.

Lang, H. G., & Albertini, J. A. (2001). Construction of meaning in the authentic science writing of deaf students. *Journal of Deaf Studies and Deaf Education, 6*(4), 258–284.

Lederberg, A. R., Prezbindowski, A. K., & Spencer, P. E. (2000). Word-learning skills of deaf preschoolers: The development of novel mapping and rapid word-learning strategies. *Child Development, 71*(6), 1571–1585.

Leybaert, J. (1993). Reading in the deaf: The roles of phonological codes. In Marschark & M. D. Clark (Eds.), *Psychological perspectives on deafness* (pp. 269–309). Hillsdale, NJ: Erlbaum.

Leybaert, J. (1998). Effects of phonetically augmented lipspeech on the development of phonological representations in deaf children. In M. Marsschark & M. D. Clark (Eds.), *Psychological perspectives on deafness* (pp. 103–130). Mahwah, NJ: Erlbaum.

Ling, D., (n.d.). *Acoustics, audition, and speech reception: Essentials underlying the development of spoken language by children who are hearing impaired.* [Videotape]. Alexandria, VA: Auditory Verbal International.

Ling, D. (2002). *Speech and the hearing-impaired child* (2nd ed.). Washington, DC: A. G. Bell Association for the Deaf and Hard of Hearing.

Ling, D., & Ling, A. (1978). *Aural habilitation.* Washington, DC: A. G. Bell Association for the Deaf and Hard of Hearing.

Loeterman, M., Paul, P. V., & Donahue, S. (2002, February). Reading and deaf children. *Reading Online, 5*(6). Retrieved April 17, 2006, from www.readingonline.org/articles/art_index.asp?HREF=loeterman/index.html

Luetke-Stahlman, B., & Nielsen, D. (2003). The contribution of phonological awareness and receptive expressive English to the reading ability of deaf students with varying degrees of exposure to accurate English. *Journal of Deaf Studies and Deaf Education, 8*, 464–484.

McAnally, P., Rose, S., & Quigley, S. (1999). *Reading practices with deaf learners.* Austin, TX: Pro-Ed.

McConkey-Robbins, P. (1998). Two paths of auditory development for children with cochlear implants. *Loud and Clear Newsletter, 1*(1) 1–4.

Mehl, A. L., & Thomson, V. (1998). Newborn hearing screening: The great omission. *Pediatrics, 101*(1) e4.

Mehl, A. L., & Thomson, V. (2002). The Colorado newborn hearing screening project 1992–1999: On the threshold of effective population-based universal newborn hearing screening. *Pediatrics, 109*(1), e7.

Meints, K., Plunkett, K., & Harris, P. L. (1999). When does an ostrich become a bird? The role of typicality in early word comprehension. *Developmental Psychology, 35,* 1072–1078.

Meltzoff, A. N. (1999). Origins of theory of mind, cognition, and communication. *Journal of Communication Disorders, 32,* 251–269.

Metsala, J. L., & McCann, A.D., & Dacey, A.C. (1997). Children's motivations for reading. *Reading Teacher, 50*(4), 360–363.

Moog, J., & Geers, A. (1990). *Early Speech Perception (ESP) test for profoundly hearing-impaired children.* St. Louis: Central Institute for the Deaf.

Moog, J. S., & Biedenstein, J. J. (1998). *Teacher assessment of spoken language.* St. Louis, MO: The Moog Oral School.

Moog, J. S., Stein, K., Biedenstein, J, & Gustus, C. (2003). *Teaching activities for children who are deaf and hard of hearing: A practical guide for teachers.* St. Louis: The Moog Center for Deaf Education.

National Institute of Child Health and Human Development. (2002). *Report of the National Reading Panel: Teaching children to read.* Retrieved May 15, 2006, from www.nationalreadingpanel.org/Publications/subgroups.htm

National Institute on Deafness and Other Communication Disorders. (n.d.). *Speech and language development milestones.* Retrieved April 17, 2006, from www.nidcd.nih.gov/health/voice/speechandlanguage.asp

Nevins, M. E., & Chute, P. M., (1996). *Children with cochlear implants in educational settings.* San Diego: Singular Publishing.

Newport, E. L. (1991). Contrasting conceptions of the critical period for language. In S. Carey & R. Gelman (Eds.), *The Epigenesis of mind: Essays on biology and cognition.* Hillsdale, NJ: Erlbaum.

Nixon, M. (2004). Standards for acoustical environments in educational settings. *Hearing, 25*(2), 113–114.

Norris, J. A., & Hoffman, P. R. (1994). Whole language and representational theories: Helping children to build a network of associations. *Journal of Childhood Communication Disorders, 16*(1), 5–12.

Northern, J. L., & Downs, M. P. (2001). *Hearing in children* (5th ed.). Philadelphia: Lippincot Williams & Wilkins.

O'Hare, C. B. (1987). The effect of verbal labeling on tasks of visual perception: An experimental investigation. *Educational Research, 29*(3), 213–219.

Oller, D. (1978). Infant vocalizations and the development of speech. *Allied Health and Behavior Sciences, 1,* 523–549.

Owens, R., Jr. (1996.) *Language development: An introduction* (4th ed.). Needham Heights, MA: Allyn & Bacon.

Paul, P. (1998). *Literacy and deafness: The development of reading, writing, and literate thought.* Boston: Allyn & Bacon.

Peng, S., Spencer, L. J., & Tomblin, J. B. (2004). Speech intelligibility of pediatric cochlear implant recipients with seven years of device experience. *Journal of Speech Language and Hearing Research, 47*(6), 1227.

Perfetti, C. A., & Sandak, R. (2000). Reading optimally builds on spoken language. Implications for deaf readers. *Journal of Deaf Studies and Deaf Education, 5,* 32–50.

Pinker, S. (1994). *The language instinct: How the mind creates language.* New York: HarperCollins.

Pollack, D., Goldberg, D., & Caleffe-Schenck, N. (1997). *Educational audiology for the limited-hearing infant and preschooler* (3rd ed.). Springfield, IL: Charles C Thomas.

Prezbindowski, A. K., & Lederberg, A. R. (2003). Vocabulary assessment of deaf and hard-of-hearing children: From infancy through the preschool years. *Journal of Deaf Studies and Deaf Education, 7,* 330–345.

Proctor, R., Niemeyer, J. A., & Compton, M. V. (2005). Training needs of early intervention personnel working with infants and toddlers who are deaf and hard of hearing. *The Volta Review, 105*(2), 113–128.

Rhoades, E. (2000). *Motherese-parentese or strategies we employ to facilitate language learning.* Retrieved May 15, 2006, from Auditory Verbal Training-Workshops-Consultants-Mentoring Website: www.auditoryverbaltraining.com/motherese.htm

Rosenshine, B., & Meister, C. (1992). The use of scaffolds for teaching higher-level cognitive strategies. *Educational Leadership, 49*(7), 26–33.

Rossing, T. D. (1990). *The science of sound* (2nd ed.). Upper Saddle River, NJ: Pearson Education.

Ruben, R.J. (1997). A time frame of critical/sensitive periods of language development. *Acta Otlaryngologica, 117*(2), 202–205.

Sajaniemi, N., Hakamies-Blomqvist, L., Makela, J., Avellan, A., Rita, H., & von Wendt, L. (2001). Cognitive development, temperament and behavior at 2 years as indicative of language development at 4 years in pre-term infants. *Child Psychiatry & Human Development. 31*(4), 329–346.

Sass-Lehrer, M., & Bodner-Johnson, B. (2003). Early intervention: Current approaches to family-centered programming. In M. Marschark & P. Spencer (Eds.), *Oxford handbook of deaf studies, language, and education* (pp. 65–81). New York: Oxford University Press.

Schafer, G., Plunkett, K., & Harris, P. L. (1999). What's in a name? Lexical knowledge drives infants' visual preference in the absence of referential point. *Developmental Science, 2,* 187–194.

Scharer, P. L., Pinnell, G. S., Lyons, C., & Fountas, I. (2005). Becoming an engaged reader. *Educational Leadership, 63*(2), 24–29.

Schirmer, B. (2000). *Language and literacy development in children who are deaf* (2nd ed.). Boston: Allyn & Bacon.

Schirmer, B. (2003). Using verbal protocols to identify the reading strategies of students who are deaf. *Journal of Deaf Studies and Deaf Education, 8*(2), 157–170.

Schleper, D. (1997). *Reading to deaf children: Learning from deaf adults.* Washington, DC: Gallaudet University, Pre-College National Mission Programs.

Schumaker, J. B., & Sheldon, J. B. (1999). *Proficiency in the sentence writing strategy: Instructor's manual.* Lawrence: University of Kansas.

Seep, B., Glosemeyer, R., Hulce, E., Linn, M., & Aytar, P. (2000). *Classroom acoustics: A resource for creating learning environments with desirable listening conditions.* Melville, NY: American Acoustical Society.

Seikel, A. J., King, D. W., & Drumright, D. G. (2005). *Anatomy and physiology for speech, language, and hearing* (2nd ed.). San Diego: Singular Publishing Group.

Staller, S. J., Beiter, A. L., Brimacombe, J. A., Mecklenburg, D. J., & Arndt, P. (1991). Pediatric performance with the Nucleus 22-channel cochlear implant system. *American Journal of Otology, 12,* 126–136.

Stark, R. E., Ansel, B. M., & Bond, J. (1988). Are prelinguistic abilities predictive of learning disability? A follow-up study. In R. L. Masland and M. W. Masland (Eds.), *Preschool prevention of reading failure.* Parkton, MD: York Press.

Strong, C. J. (1998). *The Strong narrative assessment procedure.* Eau Claire, WI: Thinking Publications.

Tade, W. J., & Vitali, G. J. (1994). *Children's early intervention for speech-language-reading (CEI).* East Aurora, NY: Slosson Educational Publications, Inc.

Trainor, L. J., Samuel, S. S., Desjardins, R. N., & Sonnadara, R. R. (2001). Measuring temporal resolution in infants using mismatch negativity. *Neuroreport, 12*(11), 2443–2448.

Trezek, B. J., & Wang, Y. (2006). Implications of utilizing a phonics-based reading curriculum with children who are deaf or hard of hearing. *Journal of Deaf Studies and Deaf Education, 11*(2) 202–213.

Vygotsky, L. (1978). *Mind in society: The development of higher psychological processes.* Cambridge, MA: Harvard University Press.

White, K. R. (2003). The current status of EHDI programs in the United States. *Mental Retardation & Developmental Disabilities Research Reviews, 9*(2), 79–88.

Whitfield, P., & Stoddart, M. (1985). *Hearing, taste, and smell.* New York: Torstar Books.

Woodward, A., & Hoyne, K. (1999). Infants learning about words and sounds in relation to objects. *Child Development, 70*(1), 65–77.

Yoshinaga-Itano, C., & Downey, D. M. (1996). Development of school-aged deaf, hard-of-hearing, and normally hearing students' written language. *Volta Review, 98*(1), 3–7.

Yoshinaga-Itano, C., Sedey, A. L., Coulter, D. K., & Mehl, A. L. (1998). Language of early- and later-identified children with hearing loss. *Pediatrics, 102*(5), 1161–1171.

Zarrella, S. (1995). Managing communication problems of unilateral hearing loss. *ADVANCE for Speech Language Pathologists & Audiologists* (February 13, p. 12). American Speech and Hearing Association.

Index

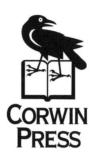

CORWIN
PRESS